Advances in Intelligent Systems and Computing

Volume 1360

The series "Advances in Intelligent Systems and Computing" contains publications on theory, applications, and design methods of Intelligent Systems and Intelligent Computing. Virtually all disciplines such as engineering, natural sciences, computer and information science, ICT, economics, business, e-commerce, environment, healthcare, life science are covered. The list of topics spans all the areas of modern intelligent systems and computing such as: computational intelligence, soft computing including neural networks, fuzzy systems, evolutionary computing and the fusion of these paradigms, social intelligence, ambient intelligence, computational neuroscience, artificial life, virtual worlds and society, cognitive science and systems, Perception and Vision, DNA and immune based systems, self-organizing and adaptive systems, e-Learning and teaching, human-centered and human-centric computing, recommender systems, intelligent control, robotics and mechatronics including human-machine teaming, knowledge-based paradigms, learning paradigms, machine ethics, intelligent data analysis, knowledge management, intelligent agents, intelligent decision making and support, intelligent network security, trust management, interactive entertainment, Web intelligence and multimedia.

The publications within "Advances in Intelligent Systems and Computing" are primarily proceedings of important conferences, symposia and congresses. They cover significant recent developments in the field, both of a foundational and applicable character. An important characteristic feature of the series is the short publication time and world-wide distribution. This permits a rapid and broad dissemination of research results.

Indexed by DBLP, INSPEC, WTI Frankfurt eG, zbMATH, Japanese Science and Technology Agency (JST).

All books published in the series are submitted for consideration in Web of Science.

More information about this series at http://www.springer.com/series/11156

Natalia Piaseczna · Magdalena Gorczowska ·
Agnieszka Łach
Editors

Innovations and Developments of Technologies in Medicine, Biology and Healthcare

Proceedings of the IEEE EMBS International Student Conference (ISC)

Springer

Editors
Natalia Piaseczna
Department of Biosensors and Processing
of Biomedical Signals
Silesian University of Technology
Zabrze, Poland

Magdalena Gorczowska
Department of Measurement and Electronics
AGH University of Technology
Kraków, Poland

Agnieszka Łach
Department of Biosensors and Processing
of Biomedical Signals
Silesian University of Technology
Zabrze, Poland

ISSN 2194-5357 ISSN 2194-5365 (electronic)
Advances in Intelligent Systems and Computing
ISBN 978-3-030-88975-3 ISBN 978-3-030-88976-0 (eBook)
https://doi.org/10.1007/978-3-030-88976-0

This Springer imprint is published by the registered company Springer Nature Switzerland AG
The registered company address is: Gewerbestrasse 11, 6330 Cham, Switzerland

Foreword

Engineering and technological innovations have significantly promoted and advanced scientific discoveries over the last few decades. These rapid innovations have increased the quality and accessibility of healthcare worldwide. Since 1952, IEEE EMBS has played a key role to highlight, promote, and translate these broad and cutting-edge emergent technologies into healthcare practices, subsequently positively impacting education and quality of life globally.

Now, there is an urgent need for biomedical engineers, clinicians, and healthcare industry leaders to work together to develop novel diagnostics and treatments. As the largest international organization that unites engineers, physicians, clinicians, healthcare leaders, and scientists to address global healthcare challenges, we strive for equal access to healthcare innovations and discoveries.

We, the IEEE Engineering in Biology and Medicine Society, will continue fostering and promoting global biomedical engineering innovations, research, and education. Our aim is to improve the lives of all humanity, as well as to increase general awareness on the impact of biomedical engineering innovations in health care, economy, and society. To achieve this, we will continue building a vibrant, global ecosystem of engineers, scientists, physicians, healthcare professionals, and industry leaders. In this ecosystem, we openly exchange ideas, disseminate our research, and share data and protocols.

To accentuate these critical emerging areas, the IEEE EMBS International Student Conference (ISC) organized by exceptional students from Silesian University of Technology (Gliwice, Poland) and AGH University of Science and Technology (Kraków, Poland) aimed to highlight and discuss how these broad and cutting-edge emergent technologies including brain initiatives, precision medicine, computational medicine, and health informatics as well as their influences and impacts on education and humanity can be translated into cutting-edge health solutions in clinics.

The ISCs provide a unique platform for scientists, engineers, and students to focus on transnational research, engineering innovations and entrepreneurship, as well as the need for a paradigm shift in engineering and science education and their impact on economic growth. Furthermore, they play an important role in the preparation of a highly qualified workforce that has a well-rounded understanding of medical and engineering concepts and is well versed in all the relevant aspects of these emerging engineering innovations for the next generation healthcare.

I was highly impressed with the scientific quality of the conference, and I wholeheartedly congratulate Ms. Agnieszka Łach, the conference chair for her exceptional leadership, and the conference advisors, Professor P Augustyniak and Professor E Tkacz, for their exemplary mentorship of the conference committee members.

March 2021

Metin Akay
President, IEEE EMBS

Preface

This book constitutes the proceeding of IEEE EMBS International Student Conference (ISC) held online in Zabrze, December 11–12, 2020. The conference was organized in cooperation between Students from Silesian University of Technology (Gliwice, Poland) and AGH University of Science and Technology (Kraków, Poland).

The International Student Conference is a special event organized by Students for Students. It creates an open environment for students, researchers, and scientists for presenting the results of their recent work and learning about new trends in biomedical engineering. The conference is an opportunity to inspire students towards an academic career and encourage them to share their research experience.

The IEEE EMBS ISC 2020 witnessed outstanding keynote presentations given by distinguished speakers:

- Professor Yasemin Akay, University of Houston, USA
  COVID-19 and the Neurological Complications
- Professor Metin Akay, University of Houston, USA
  Advanced Technologies for BRAIN
- Doctor Jean Carlos Cruz Hernandez, Massachusetts General Hospital, USA
  Transport of CSF to the retina enables remote sensing of CNS inflammation by non-invasive imaging
- Doctor Rosa H. M. Chan, City University of Hong Kong, Hong Kong
  Neural modelling: from computation to application
- Professor Daniel Razansky, University of Zurich, Switzerland
  Citius, altius, fortius–boosting image quality and speed in optoacoustic tomography
- Doctor Peter Maroti, University of Pecs, Hungary
  Additive Manufacturing Technologies in the Development of Medical Robotic Devices
- Professor Andrzej Skalski, AGH University of Science and Technology, Poland
  Mixed and Augmented Reality in Medicine

The volume consists of twenty full papers. Each submission included in this proceeding was subjected to a review process and accepted by the conference program committee. In this regard, we would like to express our great appreciation to the members of the program committee for their invaluable help in the process of creating this work. We strongly encourage the readers to contact the corresponding authors with questions and comments concerning further details in their research.

March 2021

Magdalena Gorczowska
Katarzyna Januszewska
Agnieszka Łach
Natalia Piaseczna
Juliusz Stefański
Kamil Szkaradnik

Acknowledgements

We would like to acknowledge the organizational and substantive support of Professor Piotr Augustyniak and Professor Ewaryst Tkacz (IEEE EMBS ISC 2020 Advisors). Their time and commitment made this conference an outstanding event.

We thank the student activities committee (SAC), especially their chair Jingzi An and the IEEE EMBS team for sharing the initiative and for their great technical support.

We would also like to thank the organizing committee of IEEE EMBS International Student Conference 2020 for their invaluable contribution in the success of this event.

Organization

Organizing Committee of the IEEE EMBS International Student Conference, December 2020, Poland

Conference Advisors

Piotr Augustyniak	AGH University of Science and Technology, Kraków, Poland
Ewaryst Tkacz	Silesian University of Technology, Gliwice, Poland

Conference Chair

Agnieszka Łach	Silesian University of Technology, Gliwice, Poland

Finance Chair

Juliusz Stefański	AGH University of Science and Technology, Kraków, Poland

Program Chair

Natalia Piaseczna	Silesian University of Technology, Gliwice, Poland

Technical Chair

Kamil Szkaradnik	Silesian University of Technology, Gliwice, Poland

Publication Chair

Magdalena Gorczowska	AGH University of Science and Technology, Kraków, Poland

Publicity Chair

Katarzyna Januszewska	College of Economics and Computer Science, Kraków, Poland

Scientific Committee

Contents

On the Possibility of Mathematical Unification for the Currently Applied Analysis of Actigraphic Recordings

Piotr Biegański[1,2](✉), Anna Stróż[1], Anna Duszyk[1], Marian Dovgialo[1], and Piotr Durka[1]

[1] Faculty of Physics, University of Warsaw, ul. Pasteura 5, 02-093 Warsaw, Poland
[2] Inter-faculty Individual Studies in Mathematics and Natural Sciences, , University of Warsaw, ul. Banacha 2C, 02-097 Warsaw, Poland
pbieganski@fuw.edu.pl

Abstract. Actigraphy is a simple and non-invasive method of monitoring human motor activity. While the recordings are obtained from accelerometers in a simple manner, the analysis and interpretation of the recorded data still pose a challenge, as the results presented in the literature are usually obtained with different approaches, seldom fully described or justified.

In this paper, we review two major approaches to the analysis of actigraphic data, namely, the Cole-Kripke and Sadeh families of algorithms, and show that they can be treated as special cases of a common framework. We also briefly discuss the differences between the raw acceleration data and data recorded in zero-crossing mode (ZCM).

A unifying and mathematically well-defined framework will hopefully pose a foundation for a well-defined processing of actigraphic data, allowing for efficient applications in a subset of neurological disorders in which sleep or circadian activity disturbances may be observed, where the analysis relies on parameters fitted empirically to the data from healthy subjects fails.

Keywords: Actigraphy · Cole-Kripke algorithm · Sadeh algorithm

1 Introduction

An actigraph is a wearable device, typically in the form of a wristwatch, which measures acceleration. It may be used in long-term studies to assess circadian rhythms of a subject [1], or in short-term measurements, typically conducted during night or bedtime, to assess various sleep properties, e.g. sleep quality [2]. The recordings are non-invasive, relatively unobtrusive and inexpensive, and gathered data may serve as a basis for the further diagnostic aid, particularly within sleep or circadian rhythm-related disturbances [3] (e.g. narcolepsy type

N. Piaseczna et al. (Eds.): EMBS ICS 2020, AISC 1360, pp. 1–7, 2022.
https://doi.org/10.1007/978-3-030-88976-0_1

1 in [4]), but there are also attempts to apply such method for other neuropsychological (e.g. attention deficit hyperactivity disorder (ADHD) in [5]) or neurological (e.g. in disorders of consciousness [6]) disorders. However, actigraphic data are recorded and analyzed in a variety of different ways.

In the article, we review two major approaches to the analysis of actigraphic data, namely the Cole-Kripke [7] and Sadeh ([8], version from 1989) families of algorithms, and show that they can be treated as special cases of a common framework. We also discuss methodological issues concerning different types of actigraphic data.

2 Actigraphic Data Preprocessing and Analysis

2.1 Raw Acceleration Vs. Zero-Crossing Mode

Actigraphic measurements are effectuated by accelerometers, so the starting point for all the measures are the values of acceleration (usually in units of g) along the three spatial axes. However, many of the commercially available actigraphs do not give the user a possibility to access these data, returning measurements in a type of processed form [9], e.g., above-mentioned ZCM, "time above threshold" or "digital integration" [9], or even only output classification or sleep-quantifying parameters, such as wake after sleep onset (WASO) or total sleep time (TST) [10].

Acceleration values are usually averaged over given time epochs. Such a measure is relatively invariant with respect to the length of the averaging window. However, raw acceleration data are prone to artifacts which are difficult to remove automatically, like, e.g., involuntary movements of relatively high acceleration. Therefore, instead the raw measures of acceleration, so-called "Zero-crossing mode" (ZCM) is frequently used. ZCM data are computed as the number of times the acceleration measurement changes sign in a given fixed epoch. A common practice is to set a threshold close to 0 and count the occurrences of exceeding this threshold by the absolute value of acceleration—in order to filter out low amplitude and high frequency noise.

Values of ZCM are by definition non-negative, and, unlike the acceleration, have no physical units. In theory, the maximum number of zero crossings is limited by the number of samples in the selected epoch, which is the epoch length multiplied by the sampling frequency. Therefore, theoretically, for a signal of different sampling frequency, even when using the same window length, we should scale the parameters of the analysis to a given sampling frequency. However, the frequency of human movements in the physiological range is limited by physics and physiology (3–4 Hz is the limit suggested in [1,11]), therefore it usually lies well below the sampling frequency of the actigraph.

Another convenient property of the ZCM is the natural filtering out of the high value peaks, usually related to artifacts present in the raw acceleration data. On the other hand, in the ZCM domain we lose any relation to the actual amplitude of the recorded movements. Nevertheless, a lot of approaches to the analysis of actigraphic data—including those discussed in the following sections—are based upon the ZCM.

2.2 Cole-Kripke Algorithm

Cole-Kripke algorithm, as formulated in [7], is based upon the following equation:

$$D(n) = P(W_1 E_{n-4} + W_2 E_{n-3} + W_3 E_{n-2} + W_4 E_{n-1} + W_5 E_n + W_6 E_{n+1} + W_7 E_{n+2}), \quad (1)$$

where n is the number of analyzed epoch, E_i is the value of point in the signal which is representing given epoch, W_i is the coefficient, P is the normalizing constant and $D(n)$ is the output value of a given series (single floating-point number). If $D(n) > 1$, a given epoch is classified as wake, otherwise as sleep. This algorithm is defined for ZCM data and intended to be used with one minute epoch length. For various methods of collapsing data into epochs and for non- or overlapping epochs, the values of the coefficients are different. Each time, W_i and P are derived by fitting the data to the polysomnographic (PSG) signal, which is essential for this algorithm. After the classification, additional rescoring rules—which seem to be inspired by the rules applied in scoring hypnograms (e.g. [12])—are applied, thus increasing the percentage of correct classification when compared to PSG.

Other studies (e.g., [13,14]) and commercial software packages sometimes use similar algorithms, differing in the number of epochs taken into account and the data type required as input; some of these algorithms do not apply rescoring rules after classification, so we decided to represent the Cole-Kripke algorithm family as in the following Definition 1; constant P, multiplying every W_i, can be incorporated into the W_i values.

Definition 1. *Cole-Kripke algorithm family is defined by the following equation, optionally followed by the application of rescoring rules of the form "After K epochs scored A, the next L epochs, if scored B, are rescored A".*

$$D[n] = \sum_{i=-N}^{M} W(i)x[n-i]. \quad (2)$$

Theorem 1. *Equation defining the Cole-Kripke family (2) is equivalent to a FIR filtering of order $N + M$ followed by shifting the signal by N samples and optional application of rescoring rules.*

Proof. From FIR filter definition:

$$y[n] = \sum_{i=0}^{K} b(i)x[n-i]. \quad (3)$$

After changing the indexes in the sum, so that $K - N = M$, we obtain:

$$y[n] = \sum_{i=-N}^{M} b(i+N)x[n-i-N]. \quad (4)$$

After moving the whole signal by N samples and defining $W(i) = b(i+N)$ we obtain:

$$D[n] = y[n+N] = \sum_{i=-N}^{M} W(i)x[n-i]. \tag{5}$$

This equation is equivalent to smoothing the input signal with a moving average (MA) filter. Rescoring rules (applied after thresholding) can be viewed as a nonlinear smoothing of the signal, especially when considering activity spikes.

If we think about a short period classified as A, which is in between considerably longer periods classified as B, a rescoring rule of the form given in Definition 1 will, depending on the length of this peak, either shorten it, or eliminate it by rescoring A as B. Therefore, we can treat these rescoring rules as nonlinear smoothing. Lastly, we should note that moving the signal by a few samples (which occurs after the application of the FIR filtering in Cole-Kripke algorithm) is irrelevant to further investigation, so we treat Cole-Kripke algorithm family as an ordinary FIR filter with optional rescoring rules.

2.3 Sadeh Algorithm[1]

Sadeh algorithm, as formulated by Sadeh et al. in 1989 [8] is, just like the Cole-Kripke algorithm, intended to be used on ZCM data gathered during bedtime. Similarly, the weights (C_i) assigned to each element in the following Eq. (6), which defines this algorithm, are derived empirically by fitting the data to the sleep/wake classification derived from PSG recordings. It is based upon the following equation

$$PS(n) = C_1 + C_2X_n + C_3S_{-5} + C_4S_9 + C_5M_2 + C_6S_{-2}, \tag{6}$$

where X_n is the value of n-th epoch, S_{-5} is the standard deviation of prior 5 epochs, S_9 is the standard deviation of the following 9 epochs, M_2 is the minimal value of the following 2 epochs, S_{-2} is the standard deviation of prior 2 epochs and $PS(n)$ is output value of given series (single floating-point number). If $PS(n)$ is positive, then the epoch n is classified as sleep, otherwise it is classified as wake. It is also worth noting that this particular form of Eq. (6) was derived using discriminant analysis, and its physiological interpretation is not discussed by the authors.

Just like in the case of Cole-Kripke algorithm, we may write down an equation defining the Sadeh algorithm family. For the sake of clarity, we rename the constants given in the original formulation of the algorithm as follows: $D := C_1$, $C'(i-2) := C_i$ for $i \geq 3$, and also n-th sample from input signal we change from X_n (original formulation in [8]) to $x[n]$. We also note that that the component C_2X_n is in fact a FIR filter of order 0.

[1] Here We Describe an Early Version of Sadeh Algorithm from 1989, Not to Be Confused with the Work [15] from 1994

Definition 2. *Sadeh algorithm family is defined by the following equation:*

$$PS[n] = \sum_{i=0}^{N} W(i)x[n-i] + \sum_{i=1}^{K} C'(i)\phi_i[n] + D, \tag{7}$$

where x is an input signal, W is vector defining FIR filter (together with order N), $\phi_i[n]$ is some nonlinear filter applied to epoch n. By some nonlinear filter applied to the epoch n we understand that while this filter may take into account also different points of input vector than n (e.g. S_{-5} from Eq. (6)), the output of this filter will be on the position n in output vector PS and also this filter is in a sense defined for epoch n (e.g. S_{-5} from Eq. (6)).

The first component of this equation is responsible for smoothing the signal. Now we will argue that the components S_i from (6) are similar in function to the rescoring rules used in the Cole-Kripke algorithm family.

As mentioned, this algorithm is intended to be used on ZCM data gathered during bedtime, hence we expect that the signal from a healthy subject should mostly consist of low values with occasional high values indicating wake. This kind of properties can be found in ZCM data, as presented, e.g., in [8]. In the original formulation, as in [8], $C_3, C_4, C_6 > 0$ and $C_2, C_5 < 0$, so if we treat sleep as the desired state, we see that model is rewarded by high standard deviation (and of course penalised by high value of ZCM signal). The only case, in which the variance of such a signal is high, is when a short peak of high values is surrounded by consistently low values (or vice versa, which seems to not be the case in real data). In other words, if a short peak of high values is encountered in the data, the model will penalise high values of input data and reward shorter peaks. This is clearly of similar function as the rescoring rules in the Cole-Kripke algorithm family. The mentioned interpretation of variance filters is further supported by other researches, in which variance filtering is used to detect edges (e.g. [16]), as well as by similarity to rescoring rules.

3 A Unifying Formulation of Processing

Discussed above algorithm families share some common properties: both are to an extent empirical, both are designed to be used on ZCM data gathered during bedtime, and both are mostly centered around smoothing the signal by linear and nonlinear filtering. We propose a unified description of these two families in a form given in the following Definition 3.

Definition 3. *Unified description of Cole-Kripke and Sadeh algorithm families is given by equation:*

$$PS[n] = \sum_{i=0}^{N} W(i)x[n-i] + \sum_{i=1}^{M} C'(i)\phi_i[n] + D \tag{8}$$

followed by an optional application of rescoring rules of the form "After K epochs scored A, the next L epochs, if scored B, are rescored A".

In equation above $N \geq 0$ and stands for order of FIR filter and $M \geq 1$. Equation (8) is actually equivalent to Eq. (6) from the Sadeh algorithm and Eq. (2) can be derived by setting $C'(i)$ and D to zero. However, Cole-Kripke algorithm cannot be treated as a special case of the Sadeh algorithms, because of the extra rescoring rules present in the Cole-Kripke case. Furthermore, the rescoring rules cannot be treated as ϕ_i, because the order of transformations is in this case important. Using the rescoring rules as ϕ_i is by definition impossible, as ϕ_i is applied to a signal that is not scored yet.

Additionally, the order of FIR filtering, used in the analysis of actigraphic data ranges from 0 as in [8] to over a hundred, as in [17]. Finally, the nonlinear components ϕ_i may take significantly different forms, as for example in [15]. These issues suggest that the proposed unified formulation (8) is just the first attempt on the way to clarifying the workings and differences between different algorithms, commonly applied in the analysis of actigraphic data.

4 Summary

We have shown that the two common approaches to actigraphic signal analysis can be described in one equation, and such description clearly indicates some basic assumptions of both of these algorithms. However, we have to emphasize that there are also other—at first glance similar—algorithms, which were not included in the current attempt, because of a slightly more complicated formula [18] or lesser popularity [12].

Such a common view of mathematical properties may highlight the similarities and differences between methods used in different studies. Nevertheless, it must be clearly stated that all these approaches share inherent problems related to the empirical choice of their parameters. For example, Cole et al. [7] underlined the fact that their algorithm was designed for a specific device, and that there is a need to adapt them, as the actigraphic hardware may differ (e.g. built-in transducers). Furthermore, the coefficients of both discussed models were derived empirically, using specific datasets—therefore, such algorithms cannot be treated as universally applicable [6].

The meaning of the "unification" proposed in this preliminary study was by no means equivalent to writing down all the known approaches in one long equation; on the contrary, we wanted to highlight common elements (i.e., the presence of a type of FIR filtering and smoothing) in some of the most popular approaches, hoping to facilitate a more concrete and concise description of methods applied in the field. Apart from this, the interpretation of significant parts of the discussed algorithms as FIR filters may also facilitate a future direct comparison of their properties in a standard framework of signal analysis.

References

1. Ancoli-Israel, S., Cole, R., Alessi, C., Chambers, M., Moorcroft, W., Pollak, C.P.: The role of actigraphy in the study of sleep and circadian rhythms. Sleep **26**(3), 342–392 (2003)

2. Berger, A.M., Wielgus, K.K., Young-McCaughan, S., Fischer, P., Farr, L., Lee, K.A.: Methodological challenges when using actigraphy in research. J. Pain Sympt. Manag. **36**(2), 191–199 (2008)
3. Smith, M.T., et al.: Use of actigraphy for the evaluation of sleep disorders and circadian rhythm sleep-wake disorders: An American Academy of Sleep Medicine Clinical Practice Guideline. J. Clin. Sleep. Med. **14**(7), 1231–1237 (2018)
4. Leger, D., et al.: Using actigraphy to assess sleep and wake rhythms of narcolepsy type 1 patients: a comparison with primary insomniacs and healthy controls. Sleep Medi. **52**, 88–91 (2018)
5. Ochab, J.K., et al.: Classifying attention deficit hyperactivity disorder in children with non-linearities in actigraphy. arXiv preprint arXiv:1902.03530 (2019)
6. Cruse, D., et al.: Actigraphy assessments of circadian sleep-wake cycles in the Vegetative and minimally conscious states [published correction appears in BMC Med. 16(1) (2018)]. BMC Med. **11**(18) (2013)
7. Cole, R.J., Kripke, D.F., Gruen, W., Mullaney, D.J., Gillin, J.C.: Automatic sleep/wake identification from wrist activity. Sleep **15**(5), 461–469 (1992)
8. Sadeh, A., Alster, J., Urbach, D., Lavie, P.: Actigraphically-based automatic bedtime sleep-wake scoring: Validity and clinical applications. J. Ambul. Monit. **2**, 209–216 (1989)
9. Calogiuri, G., Weydahl, A., Carandente, F.: Methodological issues for studying the rest-activity cycle and sleep disturbances: a chronobiological approach using actigraphy data. Biol. Res. Nurs. **15**(1), 5–12 (2013)
10. Conley, S., et al.: Agreement between actigraphic and polysomnographic measures of sleep in adults with and without chronic conditions: a systematic review and meta-analysis. Sleep Med. Rev. **46**, 151–160 (2019)
11. Redmond, D.P., Hegge, F.W.: The design of human activity monitors. In: Scheving, L.E., Halberg, F., Ehret, C.F. (eds.) Chronobiotechnology and Chronobiological Engineering. NATO ASI Series (Applied Science Institutes Series), vol 120, pp. 202-215. Springer, Dordrech (1987)
12. Webster, J., Kripke, F., Messin, S., Mullaney, D., Wyborney, G.: An activity-based sleep monitor system for ambulatory use. Sleep **5**(4), 389–399 (1982)
13. Christakis, Y., Mahadevan, N., Patel, S.: SleepPy: a python package for sleep analysis from accelerometer data. J. Open Sour. Softw. **4**(44), 1663 (2019)
14. Nazaki, K., et al.: Validity of an algorithm for determining sleep/wake states using a new actigraph. J. Physiol. Anthropol. **33**, 31 (2014)
15. Sadeh, A., Sharkey, K.M., Carskadon, M.A.: Activity-based sleep-wake identification: an empirical test of methodological issues. Sleep. **17**(3), 201–207 (1994)
16. Fabijańska, A.: Variance filter for edge detection and edge-based image segmentation. In: 2011 Proceedings of 7th International Conference on Perspective Technologies and Methods in MEMS Design, MEMSTECH (2011)
17. Fuster G., Breso, A., Miranda, J.M., Garcia-Gomez, J.M.: Atigraphy pattern analysis for outpatient monitoring. Methods Mol. Biol. (Clifton, N.J.), **1246**, pp. 3–17 (2015)
18. Sazonov, E., Sazonova, N., Schuckers, S., Neuman, M., CHIME study group: Activity-based sleep-wake identification in infants. Physiol.l Measur. **25**, 1291 (2004)

Nuclei Detection in Images of Hematoxylin and Eosin-Stained Tissues Using Normalization of Value Channel in HSV Color Space

Kuba Chrobociński(✉)

Department of Biocybernetics and Biomedical Engineering, AGH University of Science and Technology, A. Mickiewicza 30 Avenue, 30–059 Kraków, Poland
chrobocinski@student.agh.edu.pl

Abstract. Hematoxylin and Eosin staining is one of the most popular techniques used in histopathology, but it has not been yet fully automated. Nuclei segmentation still stays unsolved among the problems that present themselves. Many approaches have been developed, but they often focus on the tissue of one organ. Standardizing the method of segmentation and detection of HE stained tissue samples could provide benefits for histopathologists, because even currently they have to perform this kind of time-consuming tasks. This article presents an approach to nuclei segmentation and detection using the transfer from RGB color space to HSV and normalization of Value channel. It also presents the results of different methods of binarization after normalizing Value channel.

Keywords: Color normalization · Hematoxylin · Eosin · Nuclei segmentation · HSV

1 Introduction

Hematoxylin and Eosin staining is one of the most popular techniques in histopathology [1], but it has not been yet fully automated. Most algorithms focus on images of tissues that originate from one organ. Another problem is the unstandardized staining protocols, which present problems that can be difficult to overcome when developing nuclei segmentation algorithms. Standardizing the methods of segmentation and detection of nuclei in H&E-stained tissue samples could provide benefits for histopathologists because they still have to perform these time-consuming tasks manually in order to provide precise outlines of nuclei [2].

This article presents an approach to nuclei segmentation and detection that could be used to provide good results for images from various organs, regardless of the differences in staining protocols between different laboratories. This

N. Piaseczna et al. (Eds.): EMBS ICS 2020, AISC 1360, pp. 8–17, 2022.
https://doi.org/10.1007/978-3-030-88976-0_2

algorithm uses the transfer of the image from RGB color space to HSV and normalization of the *Value* channel. It also presents the results of different binarization methods after normalizing the *Value* channel. The algorithm presented in this abstract is inspired by methods and observations presented in [3–8].

2 Materials and Methods

2.1 Used Data

The algorithm was developed and tested using a dataset containing 30 images of H&E-stained tissues obtained from different organs, including the stomach, bladder, prostate, kidney, liver, breast, and colon; also used were 30 corresponding hand-made segmentations, and 30 outlines of these segmentations. The dataset was downloaded from [9].

A great variety in the shape and size of the nuclei can be observed; this is related to the origins of these images. Moreover, a wide range of colors can be noticed in the stained tissues.

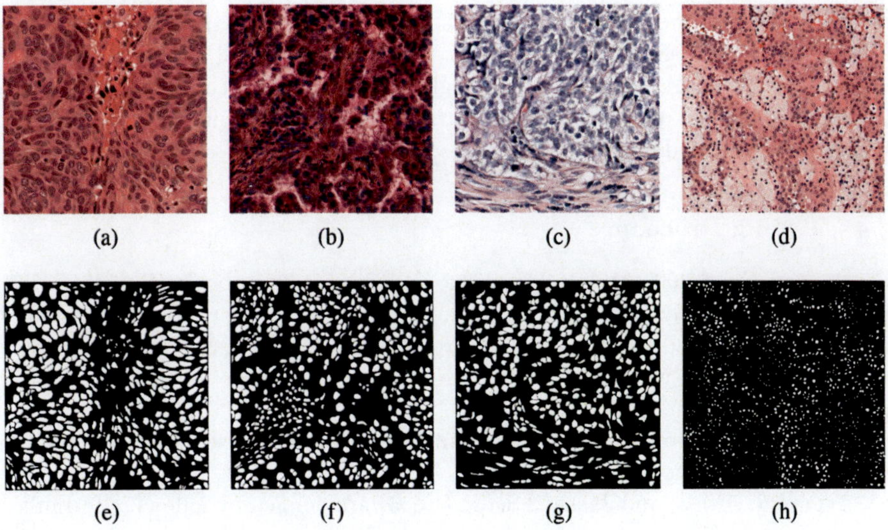

Fig. 1. Examples of original images with their corresponding handmade segmentations.

2.2 Algorithm for Nuclei Detection

Normalization. After being loaded, an image is transferred from RGB to HSV color space using a function implemented in sckit-image [10]. After transformation, the *Value* channel is extracted, then normalization is carried out using Eq. (1), as described in [11].

$$V' = \frac{\sigma_t}{\sigma_s}(V - \overline{V}) \quad (1)$$

Binarization. Eight different binarization algorithms were tested to determine which performs best. The tested algorithms were selected according to two criteria: the chosen algorithm was implemented in the sckit-image Python library [10], and it did not require additional parameters because this would prolong the already lengthy calculations. The following algorithms were chosen:

- Otsu method [12],
- Isodata method [13],
- Li method [14],
- Mean method [15],
- Niblack method [16],
- Sauvola method [17],
- Triangle method [18], and
- Yen method [19].

2.3 Parameter Set

In order to find the best pair of parameters, 8,000 pairs of mean and standard deviations were generated; these were chosen randomly in the range 0–1 using a function implemented in the Numpy Python library [20]. All these pairs of parameters were also tested with all eight binarization methods, which gives a total of 64,000 sets of different three parameters: mean, standard deviation and binarization method.

2.4 Testing Procedure

For each of the 8,000 pairs of parameters and every 8 methods of binarization, the accuracy and Jaccard scores for the 30 individual images were calculated using the hand-made segmentations provided in the dataset. Mean Accuracy and Jaccard scores were also calculated for each parameter set in order to find the optimal ones for all 30 images.

The functions implemented in Scikit-learn [21] were used to calculate the above-mentioned metrics.

Accuracy (Eq. 2) and Jaccard Score (Eq. 3) are defined by following formulas:

$$ACC = \frac{TP + TN}{TP + TN + FN + FP}, \tag{2}$$

$$JACC = \frac{TP}{TP + FN + FP}, \tag{3}$$

where:

- TP - True Positive,
- TN - True Negative,
- FP - False Positive,
- FN - False Negative.

Jaccard score was regarded as a more important metric, as the accuracy could give high results even with blank images because of matching backgrounds.

Functions implemented in Scikit-learn [21] were used to calculate above-mentioned metrics.

3 Results

From the described parameter set, one pair was successfully chosen as optimal for all 30 images based on the highest mean Jaccard score. The 30 sets of normalization parameters and binarization methods that gave the best results for each image were also selected.

Table 1. Images with best performing parameters and methods with their scores.

Image	Accuracy	Jaccard	Mean	Std	Binarization method	Organ of origin
TCGA-KB-A93J-01A-01-TS1	0.9049	0.7585	0.7192	0.1321	Isodata	Stomach
TCGA-RD-A8N9-01A-01-TS1	0.9072	0.7402	0.7124	0.7026	Isodata	Stomach
TCGA-18-5592-01Z-00-DX1	0.8707	0.7149	0.9995	0.9883	Li	Liver
TCGA-DK-A2I6-01A-01-TS1	0.9125	0.7107	0.7178	0.4348	Yen	Breast
TCGA-AR-A1AS-01Z-00-DX1	0.885	0.634	0.7393	0.8008	Otsu	Colon
TCGA-AY-A8YK-01A-01-TS1	0.8669	0.6083	0.8359	0.7021	Triangle	Kidney
TCGA-B0-5710-01Z-00-DX1	0.9522	0.607	0.6641	0.043	Otsu	Colon
TCGA-NH-A8F7-01A-01-TS1	0.8478	0.5896	0.7402	0.4551	Triangle	Bladder
TCGA-G2-A2EK-01A-02-TSB	0.9319	0.5836	0.6943	0.6074	Yen	Breast
TCGA-A7-A13F-01Z-00-DX1	0.9093	0.5761	0.7007	0.9067	Otsu	Liver
TCGA-21-5786-01Z-00-DX1	0.8236	0.5587	0.7803	0.2487	Otsu	Kidney
TCGA-HE-7130-01Z-00-DX1	0.8352	0.5572	0.7686	0.9629	Otsu	Kidney
TCGA-B0-5711-01Z-00-DX1	0.9367	0.5494	0.6763	0.0391	Otsu	Liver
TCGA-49-4488-01Z-00-DX1	0.8176	0.5473	0.998	0.207	Triangle	Breast
TCGA-A7-A13E-01Z-00-DX1	0.8982	0.5465	0.7119	0.4221	Yen	Kidney
TCGA-B0-5698-01Z-00-DX1	0.9373	0.5332	0.6567	0.6621	Yen	Prostate
TCGA-G9-6356-01Z-00-DX1	0.8859	0.5217	0.7217	0.9697	Otsu	Liver
TCGA-50-5931-01Z-00-DX1	0.7284	0.5013	0.9995	0.9883	Otsu	Breast
TCGA-AR-A1AK-01Z-00-DX1	0.8554	0.4969	0.751	0.687	Yen	Breast
TCGA-E2-A1B5-01Z-00-DX1	0.9141	0.4721	0.7002	0.0217	Yen	Breast
TCGA-E2-A14V-01Z-00-DX1	0.8606	0.4647	0.7402	0.4551	Otsu	Liver
TCGA-21-5784-01Z-00-DX1	0.904	0.4564	0.6797	0.5459	Otsu	Liver
TCGA-38-6178-01Z-00-DX1	0.8365	0.4524	0.7915	0.9419	Yen	Kidney
TCGA-HE-7128-01Z-00-DX1	0.9122	0.4505	0.6973	0.9883	Otsu	Kidney
TCGA-HE-7129-01Z-00-DX1	0.8365	0.4256	0.7163	0.7622	Otsu	Prostate
TCGA-G9-6362-01Z-00-DX1	0.7813	0.421	0.7686	0.9629	Otsu	Prostate
TCGA-G9-6336-01Z-00-DX1	0.7316	0.405	0.7974	0.5659	Otsu	Prostate
TCGA-CH-5767-01Z-00-DX1	0.811	0.36	0.7183	0.9619	Otsu	Prostate
TCGA-G9-6348-01Z-00-DX1	0.81	0.3597	0.7339	0.0478	Otsu	Prostate
TCGA-G9-6363-01Z-00-DX1	0.7799	0.3443	0.7168	0.2866	Li	Prostate

In Fig. 2, four images are presented whose results are compared with the hand-made segmentations. Black pixels are True Positives, Blue are False Negatives, and Red are False Positives. It should be noted that the hand-made

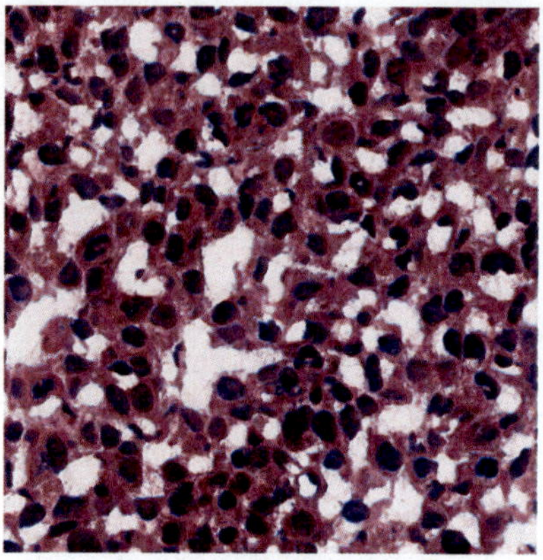

(a) TCGA-DK-A2I6-01A-01-TS1

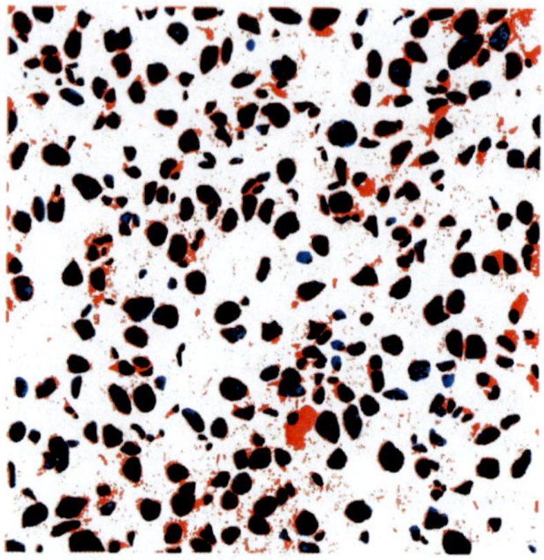

(b) Compared segmentations of TCGA-DK-A2I6-01A-01-TS1

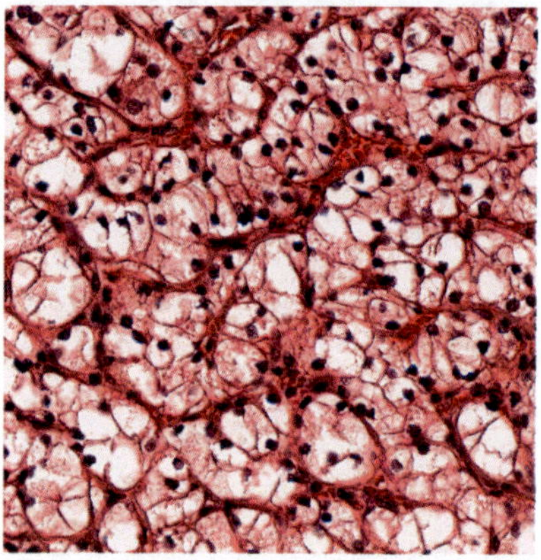

(c) TCGA-B0-5698-01Z-00-DX1

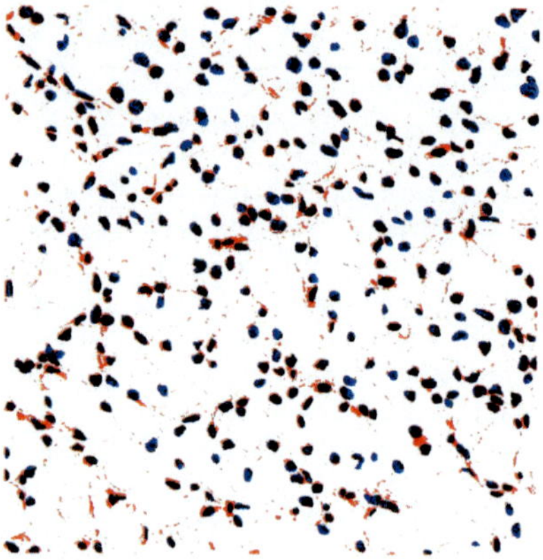

(d) Compared segmentations of TCGA-B0-5698-01Z-00-DX1

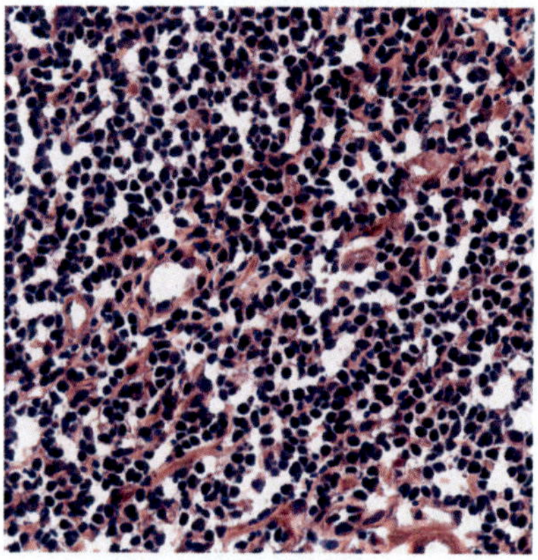

(e) TCGA-KB-A93J-01A-01-TS1

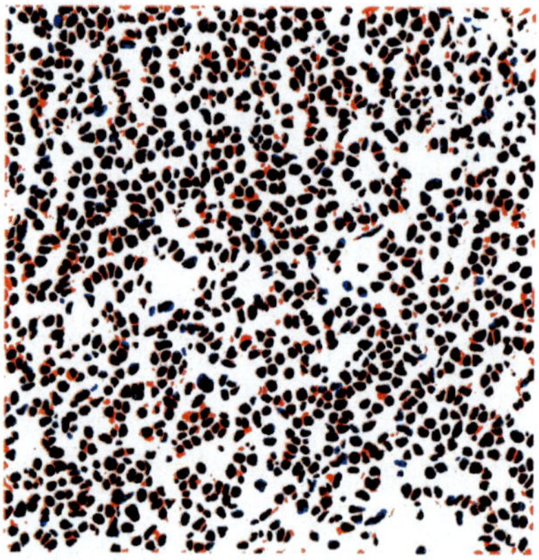

(f) Compared segmentations of TCGA-KB-A93J-01A-01-TS1

Fig. 2. Example original images with results compared with handmade segmentations (Black pixels - TP, Blue pixels - FN, Red pixels - FP).

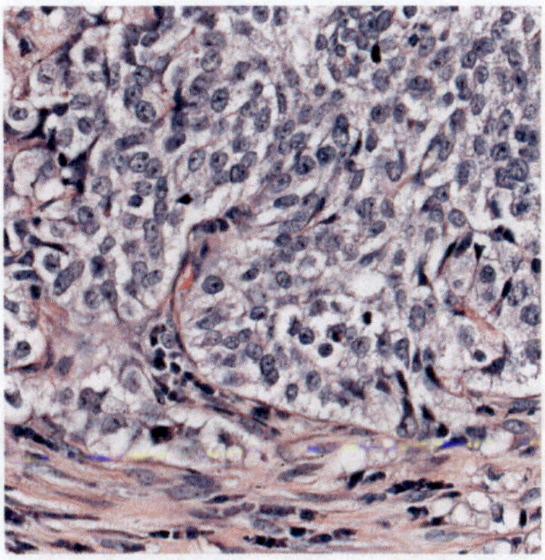

(g) TCGA-21-5786-01Z-00-DX1

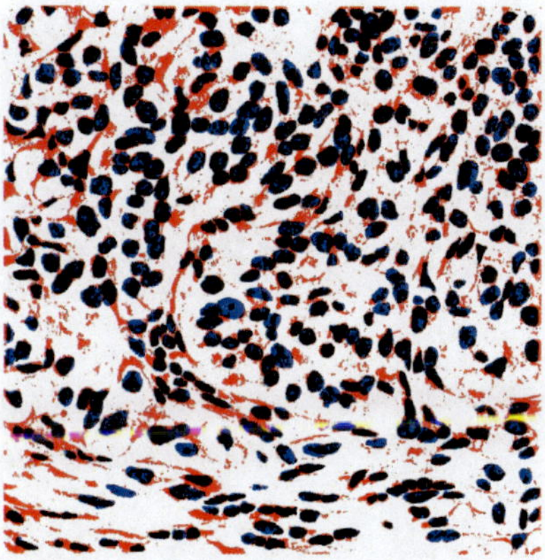

(h) Compared segmentations of TCGA-21-5786-01Z-00-DX1

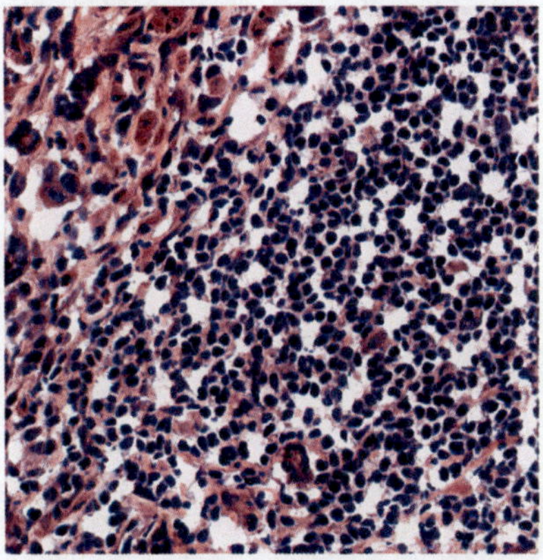

(i) TCGA-RD-A8N9-01A-01-TS1

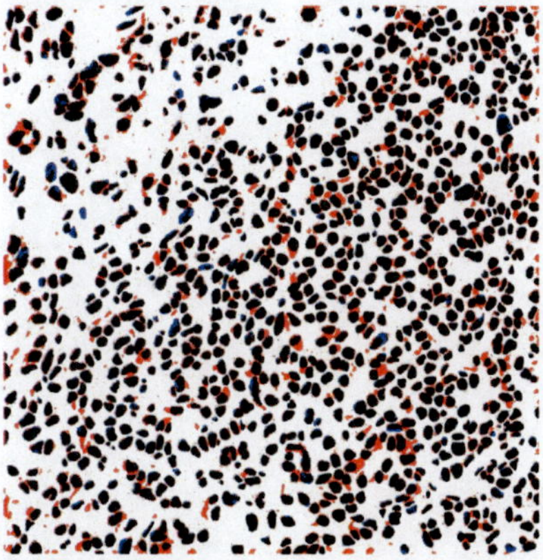

(j) Compared segmentations of TCGA-RD-A8N9-01A-01-TS1

Fig. 2. (*continued*)

segmentations do not include some of the smaller nuclei and some that are located close to the borders of the images.

The importance of the normalization procedure can be seen by comparing the value channels, inverted value channels, and normalized value channels of the images, as seen on Fig. 3.

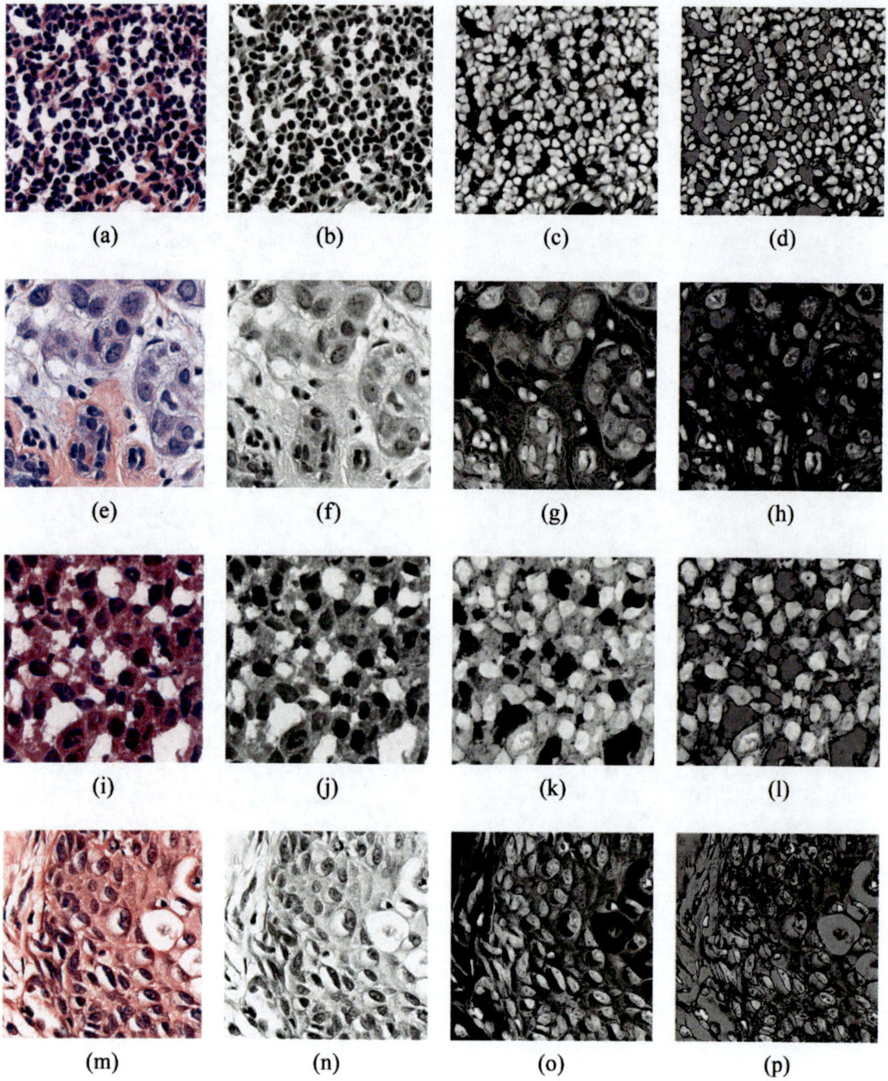

Fig. 3. Comparison of original images, their value channels, inverted Value channels and value channels after normalization.

In best-to-worst order, the three best-performing (according to the mean of the best scores among all images) binarization methods were Otsu, Isodata, and Yen (Fig. 4).

Figure 5 shows which image and which binarization method gave the best results.

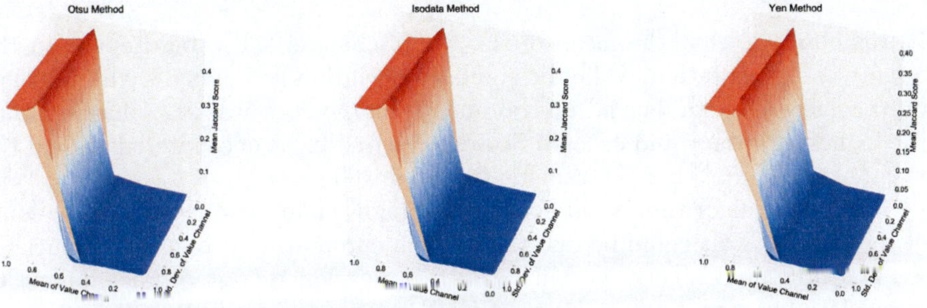

Fig. 4. Parameter spaces for three best binarization methods.

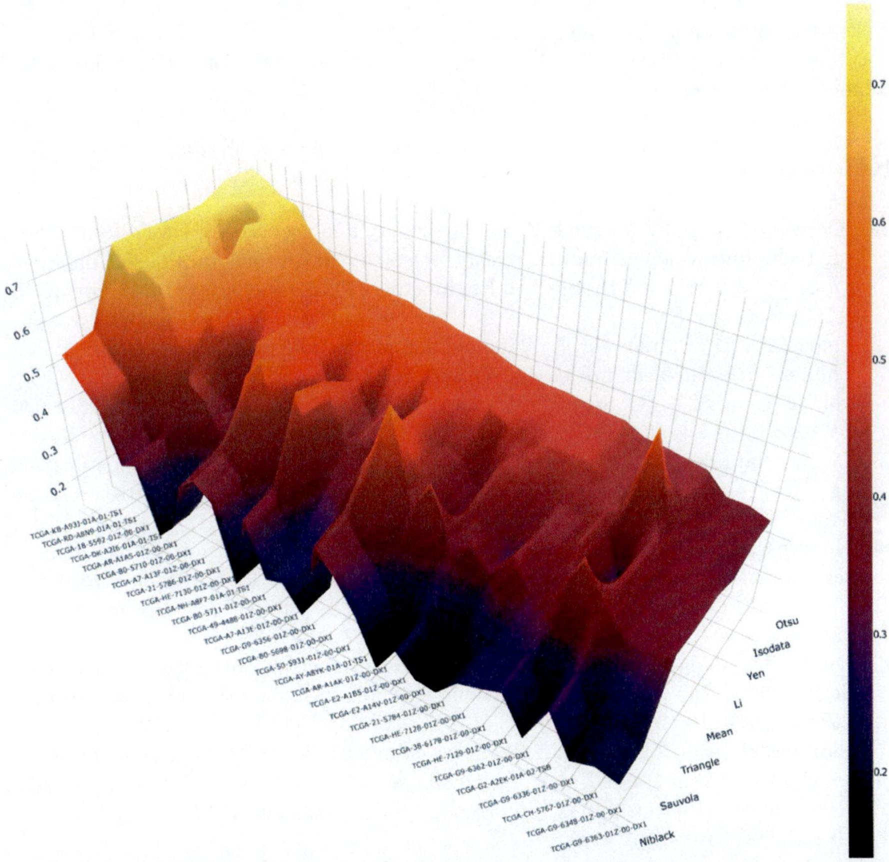

Fig. 5. Best Jaccard score for images with different binarization methods.

4 Discussion and Conclusions

It was observed that the mean of the *Value* channel had a big impact on the quality of segmentation, while the standard deviation had only a slight influence on the Jaccard score. For all images and all methods, it was also observed that the highest accuracy and Jaccard Scores appeared to be encountered around the mean of the *Value* channel, ranging from 0.6 to 0.8.

The tested algorithm could not produce high-quality segmentations for some of the images. This could be due to the open chromatin in some of the nuclei.

The presented algorithm will be further developed, tested, and applied to other datasets containing imgages of H&E stained tissues. Either changing the binarization method from thresholding to a more effective method or exploring different window sizes for Niblack and Sauvola method is considered.

Using texture analysis is considered to help segment nuclei affected by open chromatin [22].

Acknowledgement. This publication was funded by AGH University of Science and Technology, Faculty of Electrical Engineering, Automatics, Computer Science and Biomedical Engineering.

References

1. Kłeczek, P., Mól, S., Jaworek-Korjakowska, J.: The accuracy of H&E stain unmixing techniques when estimating relative stain concentrations. In: Polish Conference on Biocybernetics and Biomedical Engineering (PCBBE 2017), vol. 647, pp. 87–97. AISC, Springer (2017)
2. Dudzińska, D., Piórkowski, A.: Tissue differentiation based on classification of morphometric features of nuclei. In: Florez, H., Misra, S. (eds.) ICAI 2020. CCIS, vol. 1277, pp. 420–432. Springer, Cham (2020). https://doi.org/10.1007/978-3-030-61702-8_29
3. Li, X., Plataniotis, K.N.: A complete color normalization approach to histopathology images using color cues computed from saturation-weighted statistics. IEEE Trans. Biomed. Eng. **62**(7), 1862–1873 (2015)
4. Nurzynska, K.: Optimal parameter search for colour normalization aiding cell nuclei segmentation. In: Kozielski, S., Mrozek, D., Kasprowski, P., Małysiak-Mrozek, B., Kostrzewa, D. (eds.) BDAS 2018. CCIS, vol. 928, pp. 349–360. Springer, Cham (2018). https://doi.org/10.1007/978-3-319-99987-6_27
5. Onder, D., Zengin, S., Sarioglu, S.: A review on color normalization and color deconvolution methods in histopathology. Appl. Immunohistoche. Mol. Morphol. **22**(10), 713–719 (2014)
6. Piórkowski, A.: Color normalization-based nuclei detection in images of hematoxylin and Eosin-stained multi organ tissues. In: Choraś, M., Choraś, R.S. (eds.) IP&C 2019. AISC, vol. 1062, pp. 57–64. Springer, Cham (2020). https://doi.org/10.1007/978-3-030-31254-1_8
7. Piórkowski, A., Gertych, A.: Color normalization approach to adjust nuclei segmentation in images of hematoxylin and eosin stained tissue. In: Pietka, E., Badura, P., Kawa, J., Wieclawek, W. (eds.) ITIB 2018. AISC, vol. 762, pp. 393–406. Springer, Cham (2019). https://doi.org/10.1007/978-3-319-91211-0_35

8. Roy, S., Kumar Jain, A., Lal, S., Kini, J.: A study about color normalization methods for histopathology images. Micron **114**, 42–61 (2018)
9. Kumar, N., Verma, R., Sharma, S., Bhargava, S., Vahadane, A., Sethi, A.: A dataset and a technique for generalized nuclear segmentation for computational pathology. IEEE Trans. Med. Imag. **36**(7), 1550–1560 (2017)
10. van der Walt, S., et al.: The scikit-image contributors: scikit-image: image processing in Python. Peer J. **2**, e453 (2014). https://doi.org/10.7717/peerj.453
11. Reinhard, E., Adhikhmin, M., Gooch, B., Shirley, P.: Color transfer between images. IEEE Comput. Graph. Appl. **21**(5), 34–41 (2001)
12. Otsu, N.: A threshold selection method from gray-level histograms. Automatica **11**(285–296), 23–27 (1975)
13. Ridler, T., Calvard, S., et al.: Picture thresholding using an iterative selection method. IEEE Trans. Syst. Man. Cybern. **8**(8), 630–632 (1978)
14. Li, C., Tam, P.: An iterative algorithm for minimum cross entropy thresholding. Patt. Recogn. Lett. **19**(8), 771–776 (1998). https://doi.org/10.1016/S0167-8655(98)00057-9,www.sciencedirect.com/science/article/pii/S0167865598000579
15. Glasbey, C.A.: An analysis of histogram-based thresholding algorithms. CVGIP: Graph. Model. Image Process. **55**(6), 532–537 (1993)
16. Niblack, W.: An introduction to digital image processing. Graphical Models and Image Processing, Strandberg Publishing Company, Birkeroed (1986)
17. Sauvola, J., Pietikäinen, M.: Adaptive document image binarization. Patt. Recogn. **33**(2), 225–236 (2000)
18. Zack, G.W., Rogers, W.E., Latt, S.A.: Automatic measurement of sister chromatid exchange frequency. J. Histochem. Cytochem. **25**(7), 741–753 (1977). https://doi.org/10.1177/25.7.70454
19. Yen, J.-C., Chang, F.-J., Chang, S.: A new criterion for automatic multilevel thresholding. IEEE Trans. Image Process. **4**(3), 370–378 (1995). https://doi.org/10.1109/83.366472
20. Harris, C.R., et al.: Array programming with NumPy. Nature **585**(7825), 357–362 (2020). https://doi.org/10.1038/s41586-020-2649-2
21. Pedregosa, F., et al.: Scikit-learn: machine learning in python. J. Mach. Learn. Res. **12**, 2825–2830 (2011)
22. Jeleń, Ł: Texture description for classification of fine needle aspirates. In: Korbicz, J., Maniewski, R., Patan, K., Kowal, M. (eds.) PCBEE 2019. AISC, vol. 1033, pp. 107–116. Springer, Cham (2020). https://doi.org/10.1007/978-3-030-29885-2_10

Predicting Molecule Toxicity Using Deep Learning

Konrad M. Duraj(✉) and Natalia J. Piaseczna

Department of Biosensors and Processing of Biomedical Signals, Faculty of Biomedical Engineering, Silesian University of Technology, Roosevelta 40, Zabrze 41-800, Poland
konrad.duraj@polsl.pl

Abstract. Knowledge about certain features of molecules is crucial in many fields such as drug design. Toxicity of a compound gives information on the degree to which it can be harmful to a living organism. Experimental evaluation of a molecule's toxicity requires specialised staff and equipment and generates high costs. Deep learning is a tool used in many fields and can also be helpful in the case of predicting the molecule's toxicity. For the dataset we used a free database called 'SMILES Toxicity' which is available on kaggle. This dataset consists of 6698 non-toxic molecules and 964 toxic ones. Its imbalance creates the problem called 'overfitting'. In this article, we describe several methods for overcoming the overfitting problem. We developed two models with well-balanced true positives to false positives ratio. With the first model, we achieved 96% accuracy on the training set, 89% on the validation set and 65% on the test set. The second model scored the following values of accuracy: 80% on the training set, 78% on the validation set and 77% on the test set.

Keywords: Toxicity prediction · SMILES · Deep learning

1 Introduction

We are being exposed to a large number of chemicals everyday - through our environment, food, medicine, etc. Knowledge about the properties of certain substances is crucial to insulate our bodies from exposition to dangerous factors. The degree to which a substance can harm an organism is called toxicity. Chemical experiments evaluating the toxicity of a substance can be expensive and time consuming. This evaluation is one of the most essential steps in the process of designing drugs [1,2].

Molecule toxicity prediction is an important area of research considering its potential in helping millions of people. Given the recent advances in the field of machine learning and especially its subfield called deep learning, we can now use these techniques to help researchers and doctors all around the world make

N. Piaseczna et al. (Eds.): EMBS ICS 2020, AISC 1360, pp. 18–25, 2022.
https://doi.org/10.1007/978-3-030-88976-0_3

better predictions and speed-up the chemical/drug development process [3]. By leveraging these methods we can now analyze the chemical structure of the molecules in the form of text, images or graphs [4].

For this project, we have developed a deep recurrent neural network which can distinguish between toxic molecules from non-toxic ones. The main objective of this work is to develop a deep learning model which will be able to distinguish between toxic and non-toxic molecules from their character-based representation. Our motivation is based on three particular aspects:

- compound toxicity prediction is a challenging and critical task in drug discovery,
- current methods are restricted by the availability of experimental facilities, their resources and access to trained personnel,
- those methods are high cost in terms of both money and time,
- creating a fast, explainable and accurate way to determine the molecule's characteristics has a potential to help millions of people.

2 Materials and Methods

2.1 Dataset

For the dataset, we used 'SMILES Toxicity' which is available on the popular data science website 'kaggle.com' [5]. It contains the molecules' names, their 'SMILE'-format representation and labels (if the molecule is toxic or non-toxic). The 'SMILE' strings are also provided in the form of one-hot-encoded vectors, which can be almost directly passed to a deep neural network model.

The SMILES (Simplified Molecular-Input Line-Entry System) are ASCII strings that describe the atoms, bonds, and connectivity of a compound in a way that is both precise and easy to store. Nevertheless, it lacks the molecule's 3D information, which may be crucial in certain tasks.

The dataset contains of:

- the training set: 6760 non-toxic molecules and 937 toxic molecules,
- the test set: 238 non-toxic molecules and 27 toxic molecules.

The problem with the aforementioned dataset is the imbalance between classes. This kind of disproportion in the dataset creates the neural network's problem called 'overfitting' - that means that we could not obtain a well-balanced model, but the one that predicts only 'non-toxic' category.

The aforementioned problem is quite common and there are several ways to overcome it. We can divide these methods into two categories: data-driven and algorithm-driven. Data-driven methods apply transformations to create new, synthetic data that would resemble the minority class. This process is called data augmentation. Algorithm-driven methods prevent overfitting by manipulating the neural network's loss function and optimization process, which helps to compensate for the unequal distribution of categories.

2.2 Model I

The first attempt to overcome the overfitting problem was to create a new training set in which we reduced the number of non-toxic elements to 4500. Additionally, we have created new instances of toxic molecules by copying the already existing ones in the dataset. As a result of this operation, we obtained 3240 toxic molecules in the training set. While conducting the experiments, we manipulated these proportions as well and chose the ones giving the most promising results. We also divided the original training set into training and validation sets. In that step, we have made the recurrent neural network actually trying to optimize by analyzing sequences of one-hot-encoded molecules. The test set remained the same so that we can objectively measure the performance of the developed model.

The created classifier is a deep, bidirectional, recurrent neural network which starts with an embedding layer to prepare the network for the sequential data format. It is followed by two bidirectional long short-term memory (LSTM) networks which are initialized with 64 and 32 cells, respectively. This model

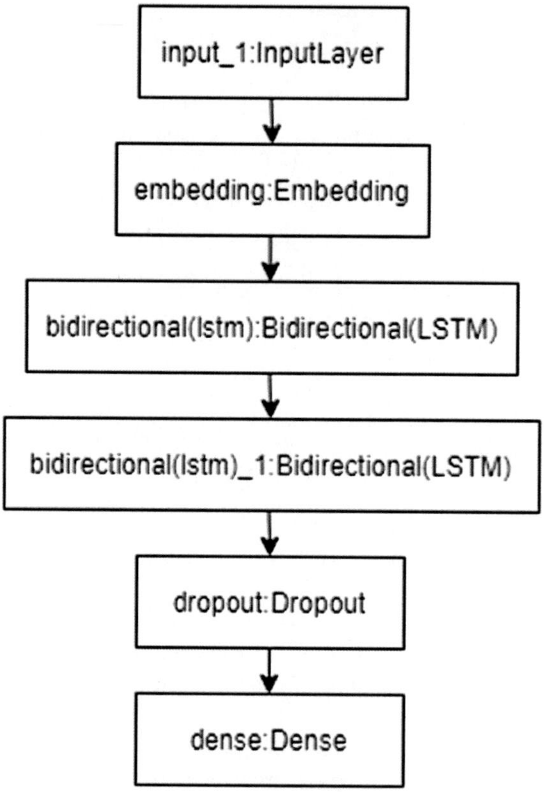

Fig. 1. Architecture of the model I

ends with a dropout layer and the final classifying layer with a single neuron activated by the sigmoid function. The architecture of the model is presented in Fig. 1.

We have decided to implement a recurrent-type network because of the character-based data type and the fact that these networks work well when analyzing time-dependent/sequential data. We have come to the conclusion that the SMILE files should also be analyzed from the beginning to the end and vice-versa because we cannot consider some part of a molecule to be the start or an end of it, that is why the recurrent units were set to learn from both these forms.

2.3 Model II

There are several methods that prevent overfitting by manipulating the neural network's loss function and optimization process. They include:

1. Loss function-based:
   - **class weighting**,
   - Mean False Error (MFE),
   - focal loss;
2. Optimization-based:
   - **cyclical/decaying learning rate**.

To create a more reliable model, we decided to apply a set of the aforementioned techniques. We chose class weighting and cyclical learning rate. These techniques help to compensate for the unequal distribution of categories.

Cyclical learning rate is a policy of learning rate adjustment that increases the learning rate of a base value in a cyclical nature. This method helps the neural network converge faster [6]. The cycles of learning rate prevents the model from getting stuck in the local minima which helps in our case to avoid the overfitting problem. Class weighting applies penalization for the misclassified examples with a certain weight. The higher the class weight, the more emphasis is put on this certain class. For our problem, we used 3.0 and 0.5 weights for toxic and non-toxic classes, respectively.

The implemented model is a hybrid of long short-term memory (LSTM) and convolution network (CNN). It contains:

- bidirectional, recurrent layer - extracting information from data in a sequential manner,
- batch normalization - regularization method,
- pooling layer - data reduction method,
- convolutional layer - extracting features in a spatial manner,
- neural layer - network's classification head.

This model was trained using the original dataset without any alterations. Total number of parameters was 329 665. The architecture of the model is presented in the Fig. 2.

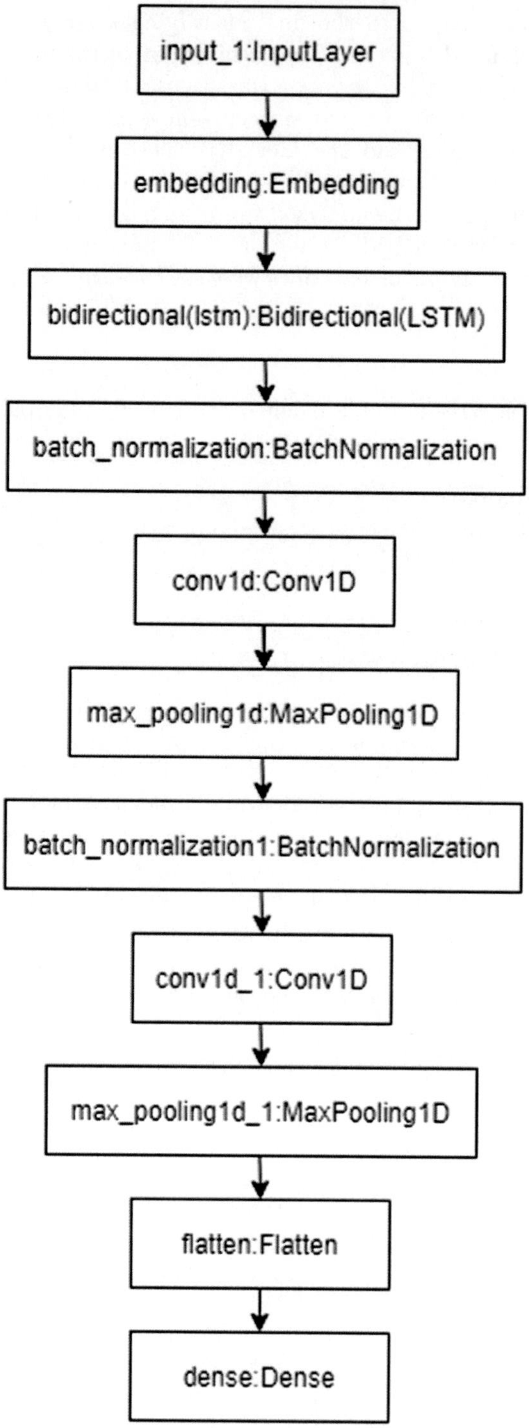

Fig. 2. Architecture of the model II

3 Results

3.1 Model I

With the first model, we have achieved 96% accuracy on the training set, 89% on the validation set (partly synthetic), and on the test set the model scored 65%. Although this model did not achieve high accuracy, it was the best-balanced one between true positives and true negatives (TP: 16; TN: 154; FP: 11; FN: 84.). Results obtained using other models (with different structure, hyper-parameters or dataset proportions) performed better on the test set (up to 81% accuracy) but they were also imbalanced between true positive and true negative predictions.

The test set contained 265 samples in which only 27 represented toxic molecules, so the model with 16 accurate identifications was almost 60% times correct. Unfortunately, this model yielded a much lower area under the ROC curve score than the second one (0.54), which is close to random prediction, which automatically disqualifies this process as the potential solution.

3.2 Model II

The model achieved 80% accuracy and 0.45 loss on the train set. On the validation set, model scored 78% accuracy and 0.49 loss. Learning curves are presented in the Fig. 3.

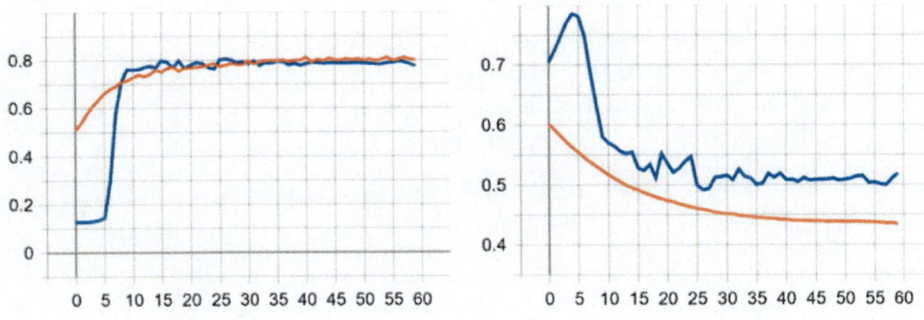

(a) Accuracy curve

(b) Loss curve

Fig. 3. Learning curves

In the Fig. 4 the metric curves are presented. Model scored:

- precision: 33% on the train set and 30% on the validation set,
- recall: 64% on the train set and 58% on the validation set,
- area under the ROC Curve: 0.8 for the train set and 0. 74 for the validation set.

The developed model was evaluated using the provided test set which contained 265 samples in total, to which 27 of them represented toxic elements and 238 non-toxic ones. Out of all the experiments, this was the model with most well-balanced true positives to true negatives ratio and most stable training process. The model yielded the following results on the test set:

- Accuracy - 77%,
- Precision - 24%,
- Recall - 52%,
- Area under ROC curve - 70%,
- Specificity - 79%,
- True positives - 14,
- True negatives - 190,
- False positives - 13,
- False negatives - 48.

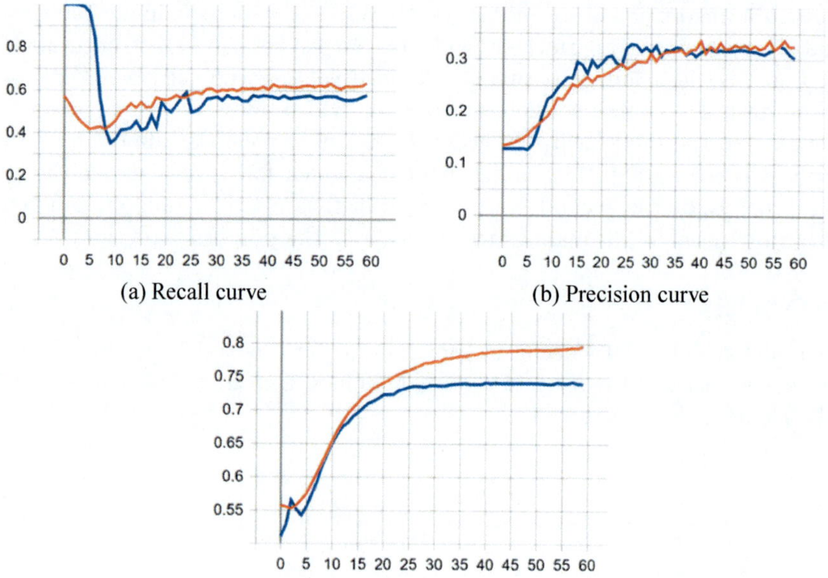

(a) Recall curve

(b) Precision curve

(c) ROC curve

Fig. 4. Metric curves

As shown in the figures above, this solution is more robust then the first one, which can be said based on the area under ROC curve score.

4 Conclusion and Discussion

We developed deep-learning models for evaluating the toxicity of molecules based on the 'SMILES Toxicity' database. In our approach, we took into account several methods for overcoming the overfitting problem. These methods included:

- extending the original toxic molecules set by replicating its instances,
- manipulating the loss function (class weighting) and optimization process (cyclical learning rate).

With these models, we achieved achieved well-balanced true positives to true negatives ratio.

Thanks to altering the dataset, the first model scored high accuracy on the train and validation set, however, this method is insufficient. On the test set, the model scored 65% accuracy – this value tells us that we did not avoid overfitting and the learning process could still be improved.

With the second model, we used the provided dataset without any alterations and yet we managed to achieve better results on the test set. The use of class weighting and cyclical learning rate allowed us to reach a more stabilized learning process which makes the model more reliable.

The use of artificial intelligence (AI) systems becomes important in many fields, especially where there is a need of expert's knowledge. Thanks to these systems, the facilities with smaller resources could use the knowledge of an expert in the form of an application. We can now train deep-learning models using the knowledge of a specialist and create a low-cost tool which will help people with making important decisions.

In the future, we plan to combine 'SMILES Toxicity' and another dataset called 'Tox21' to perform experiments using the created models on them. This way we can achieve more balanced classes with unique instances. We also plan to apply additional techniques to the imbalanced dataset problem that will stabilize the training process and explore mechanisms such as attention and active learning to create a more robust model.

References

1. Parasuraman, S.: Toxicological screening. J. Pharmacol. Pharmacotherap. **2**(2), 74–79, (2011)
2. Chen, J., Cheong, H.-H., Siu, S.W.I.: BESTox: a convolutional neural network regression model based on binary-encoded SMILES for acute oral toxicity prediction of chemical compounds. In: Martín-Vide, C., Vega-Rodríguez, M.A., Wheeler, T. (eds.) AlCoB 2020. LNCS, vol. 12099, pp. 155–166. Springer, Cham (2020). https://doi.org/10.1007/978-3-030-42266-0_12
3. Karim, A.: Toxicity prediction by multimodal deep learning. In: Ohara, K., Bai, Q. (eds.) Knowledge Management and Acquisition for Intelligent Systems, pp. 142–152. Springer International Publishing, Cham (2019)
4. Hirohara, M., Saito, Y., Koda, Y., Sato, K., Sakakibara, Y.: Convolutional neural network based on smiles representation of compounds for detecting chemical motif. In: Proceedings of the 29th International Conference on Genome Informatics (GIW 2018): Bioinformatics, vol. 19. BMC Bioinformatics (2018)
5. Fanconi, C.: Smiles toxicity, August 2019. https://www.kaggle.com/fanconic/smiles-toxicity
6. Smith, L.N.: Cyclical learning rates for training neural networks. In: 2017 IEEE Winter Conference on Applications of Computer Vision (WACV), pp. 464–472 (2017)

Adipocytokine Vaspin Stimulates the Migration Process in Different Colorectal Cancer Cell Lines

Seweryn Gałecki[1], Patrycja Niesłoń[1], Daria Kostka[1], Karol Mierzwa[1], Magdalena Węgrzyn[1], Daniel Fochtman[1], Małgorzata Adamiec[2,3](✉), Dorota Hudy[2,3], and Magdalena Skonieczna[2,3]

[1] Students' Scientific Society of Biotechnology at the Biotechnology Centre, Silesian University of Technology, Krzywoustego 8, 44-100 Gliwice, Poland

[2] Department of Systems Biology and Engineering, Silesian University of Technology, Akademicka 16, 44-100 Gliwice, Poland

[3] Biotechnology Centre, Silesian University of Technology, Krzywoustego 8, 44-100 Gliwice, Poland

malgorzata.adamiec@polsl.pl

Abstract. Colorectal carcinoma cell lines differ in invasiveness and migratory potential. Cell motility characterizes the tissue and specific resistance to genotoxic agents and protects cancer cells from the microenvironmental impact, especially from the extracellular matrix. The regulatory interactions, described as signalization loops comprised of released adipocytokines and specific for them receptors. The responses could be regulated by positive feedback, e.g., when visfatin/vaspin stimulates (up-regulates) the expression of a gene (during the incubation of cells with visfatin or vaspin), or by negative feedback when visfatin/vaspin inhibits (down-regulates) the expression of a gene. The strongest stimulation of metalloproteinases was observed under vaspin treatment in HCT116 (Duke's stage A), in LS-180 (Duke's stage B), and the weakest in HCA-2 (Duke's stage C), in comparison to the untreated control cells. Metalloproteinase gene expression in cell lines was connected to cancer invasiveness and Duke's grading system for colorectal cancers.

Keywords: Extracellular matrix · Metalloproteinases · Duke's cancer grading system · Adipocytokines · Vaspin/Visfatin stimulation

1 Introduction

In vitro cell cultures of colorectal cancer/carcinoma (CRC) cell lines differ in invasiveness and migratory potential. It is strong connected to Duke's grading system of CRC cells (Table 1). Is an estimate of the amount of penetration of a particular cancer. It is performed for diagnostic and research purposes and to determine the best method of treatment. Duke's classification including: stage A:

N. Piaseczna et al. (Eds.): EMBS ICS 2020, AISC 1360, pp. 26–32, 2022.
https://doi.org/10.1007/978-3-030-88976-0_4

limited to the mucosa; stage B1: extending into the muscularis propria but not penetrating through it; nodes not involved; stage B2: penetrating through the muscularis propria; nodes not involved; stage C1: extending into the muscularis propria but not penetrating through it; nodes involved; stage C2: penetrating through muscularis propria; nodes involved; stage D: distant metastatic spread [1].

Table 1. Characteristic and Duke's grading of colorectal cancer cell lines (based on the [7–11]).

	HCT116	$CaCo_2$	LS180	HCA2	SW116
Culture properties	ADHERENT - epithelial				
Biosafety level			1		
Tissue			COLON		
Disease	colorectal carcinoma	colorectal adenocarcinoma	colorectal adenocarcinoma	rectosigmoid adenocarcinoma	colorectal adenocarcinoma
Dukes' type	A	B	B	C	A III
Culture Conditions	Atmosphere: air, 95%; carbon dioxide (CO_2), 5% Temperature: 37 °C				Atmosphere: air, 100% Temperature: 37 °C

The cell motility characterizes the tissue and specific resistance to genotoxic agents and protects the cancer cells from the micro-environmental impact, especially from the extracellular matrix (ECM). The interaction of ECM components with cancer tissues is regulated by autocrine and paracrine signalization. Some released by adipose tissue cytokines such as vaspin, impact adipocytes, ECM component, and colorectal cancer cells of different origins. The regulatory interactions, described as signalization loops comprised of released adipocytokines and specific for the receptors. The responses could be regulated by positive feedback, e.g., when vaspin stimulates (up-regulates) the expression of a gene (during the incubation of cells with vaspin), or by negative feedback when vaspin inhibits (down-regulates) the expression of a gene. Cellular mechanisms of cancer progression started with the proliferation and migration process. The metalloproteinases (MMPs), specific enzymes necessary for the first step of ECM degradation, are required for cancer cell migration [2]. Upon adipocytokines stimulation set of MMPs are released to the cancer cells environment [3]. In colorectal cancers, regulation of metastasis process via adipocytokines, together with non-cancerous diseases of the digestive system were carefully studied [3,4].

The presented study focused on a regulatory feedback loop between stimulators visfatin or vaspin and MMPs expression, in the first step of the invasiveness pathway in colorectal cancer cell lines, in correlation to the Duke's grading system.

2 Materials and Methods

2.1 Cell Culture and Media

The experiments were done on three adherent colon cancer cell lines. HCT 116 (ATCC, cat. num.: CCL-247), HCA-2 (ECACC, cat. num.: 06061901), and LS-180 (ATCC, cat. num.: CL-187). Cells were cultivated in DMEM/F12 (PAN Biotech, cat. num.: P04-41150) supplemented with 10% FBS (Eurx, cat. num.: E5051) and 1% penicillin/streptomycin solution (Sigma-Aldrich, cat. num: P4333) at 37 °C in a humidified atmosphere with 5% of CO_2. To determine the gene expression feedback loops cells were treated for 24 h with the adipocytokine visfatin/vaspin (BioVendor) at a dose of 3 ng/ml, as was described previously [4–6].

2.2 RT-qPCR

Total RNA was isolated from cells with Total RNA mini kit (A&A Biotechnology, cat. num.: 031-100), reverse transcription was done with NG dART kit (Eurx, cat. num.: E0801) using oligo(dT) primers. Gene expression of mmp-2, mmp-9, and visfatin was determined by qPCR performed on CFX96 Touch Real-Time PCR System (BioRad), with the RT PCR Mix SYBR®A kit (A&A Biotechnology, cat. num.: 2008-1000A). Gene expression was presented as fold change to untreated control.

2.3 Statistics

All results were presented as mean +/− SD with Excel Microsoft Office 2010 software. For the correlation between stimulation of MMPs genes and Duke's grading system, the Spearman correlation coefficient was determined with Matlab XD 2019 software.

3 Results and Conclusion

MMPs gene expression in cell lines was connected to the cancer invasiveness and Dukes grading system for colorectal cancer (Table 1). The strongest stimulation of MMPs gene expression was observed under vaspin treatment in HCT116 (Duke's stage A), in LS-180 (Duke's stage B), and the weakest in HCA-2 (Duke's stage C), in comparison to the untreated controls. Such findings allow for a better understanding of the interactions of different regulators in the cancer progression and metastasis process. The cellular migration pathway, studied on the molecular level showed positive and negative feedback loops under adipocytokine treatment of colorectal carcinomas.

LS-180 cells were treated with 3 ng/ml of visfatin or vaspin for 24 h, where the expression of visfatin was determined by RT-qPCR (Fig. 1). Under both types of adipocytokine stimulation, the level of visfatin expression was up-regulated in a positive feedback loop. Visfatin is known as a cellular pathways regulator in different diseases (ovarian cancer, malignant astrocytoma, and human prostate cancer), as well as a nuclear factor in human HCT116 colorectal cancer cells [12].

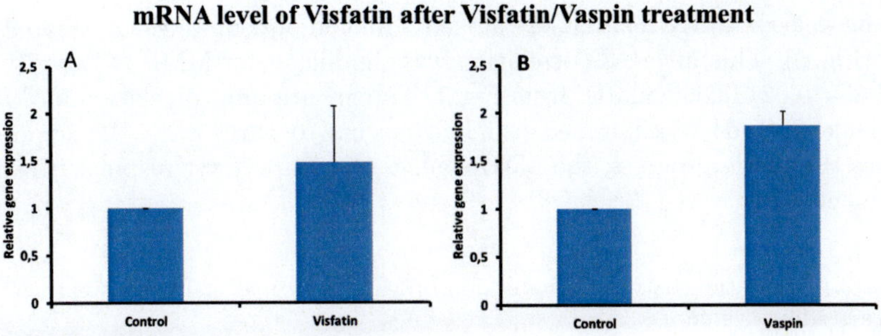

Fig. 1. Expression of visfatin in LS-180 cell line after 24 h treatment with 3 ng/ml adipocytokines – visfatin (A) or vaspin (B).

Visfatin also plays the role of an antiapoptotic factor in HCT116 and melanoma Me45 cells and protects cancer cells against oxidative stress and damage [12, 13].

Metalloproteinases, involved in the migration process, are up-regulated after adipocytokine vaspin stimulation. These findings showed that the expression of MMPs does not correlate directly with Duke's cancer grading system, as much advanced cancer type, the MMPs expression decreases (Fig. 2 and Table 2).

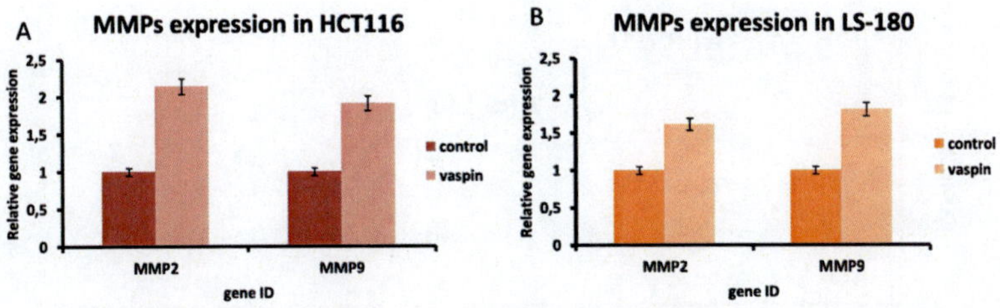

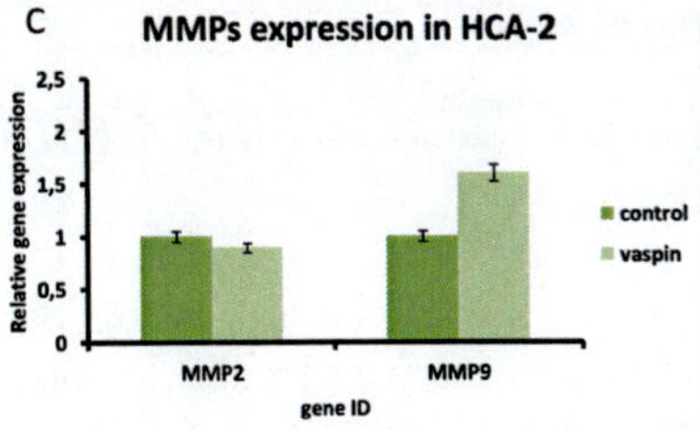

D

Relative gene expression		Ratio	
		MMP2	MMP9
HCT116 (A)	Control	1	1
	Vaspin	2.14	1.91
LS-180 (B)	Control	1	1
	Vaspin	1.61	1.81
HCA-2 (C)	Control	1	1
	Vaspin	0.89	1.60

Fig. 2. Expression of mmp-2 and mmp-9 genes in HCT 116 (A), LS-180 (B), and HCA-2 cell lines (C) 24 h after vaspin [3 ng/ml] addition. Relative gene expression presented as fold change to control (D).

The strongest stimulation of MMPs gene expression was observed under 24 h of vaspin treatment in HCT116 (Duke's stage A), in LS-180 (Duke's stage B), and the weakest in HCA-2 (Duke's stage C), in comparison to the untreated controls (Fig. 3). This inverted correlation was significant for MMP2 (Table 2) with p-value = 0,02143, calculated from Fig. 1. The Spearmann correlation for MMP2 and Duke's grade of examined cell lines seems to agree with the hypothesis that as the grade progress, the MMPs genes showed a lower response to vaspin treatment.

Table 2. Correlation between stimulation of MMP genes after vaspin treatment and Duke's grading system.

	Spearman coefficient	p-value
MMP2	**–0,79**	**0,02143**
MMP9	–0,32	0,43571

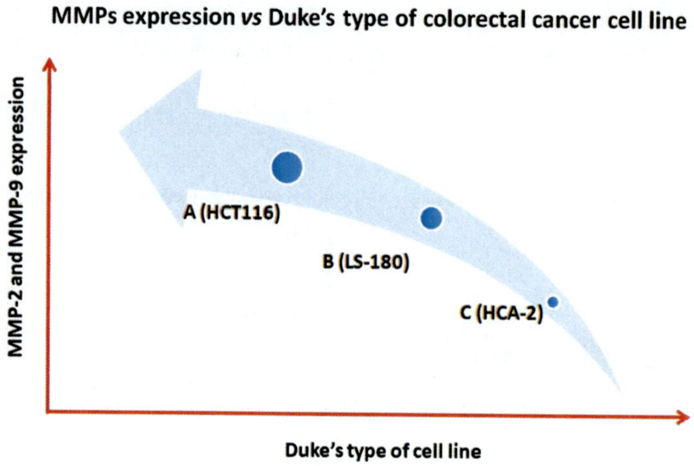

Fig. 3. Relation of MMPs expression vs Duke's grading system for CRC cells.

In concluding remarks, it was found that the cellular migration pathway, studied on the molecular level showed positive and negative feedback loops under adipocytokine treatment of colorectal carcinomas. MMPs gene expression does not correlate directly with Duke's cancer grading system, as much advanced cancer type, the MMPs expression decreases. Correlation of the MMPs production with the ability to migrate from a primary localization of tumor and metastasis via the circulatory system to novel niches is comprised and still under investigation. Extracellular matrix degradation is the hallmark of cancers of all types [14]. Invasion and metastasis are specific also for colorectal carcinoma cell lines [15], studied in live time-lapsed microscopic observations [6]. Caco-2 cells, classified as Dukes's type 2, were activated under the vaspin stimulation [IC = 2.8

ng/ml] during long term observations, the motility of the cells was enhanced in comparison to the untreated control population [6]. However, a higher concentration of the adipocytokine could be more toxic and enhanced the migratory potential of the cells. More advanced studies on the migratory potential of cells are focused on adipose tissue and adipose-derived stem cells (ADSCs) as adipocytokine producers. Adipocytes and ADSCs in obese patients suffered from non-communicable diseases (NCDs), and from CRC could be suspected for metastasis activation via cytokine storm production. Regulatory feedback loops between stimulators, such as visfatin/vaspin and targeted receptors are strongly presented upon adipocytokines stimulation. We have confirmed such connections between visfatin/vaspin and metalloproteinases in the first step of the invasiveness pathway in colorectal cancer cell lines in correlation with the Duke's grading system.

Acknowledgement. Students' Scientific Society of Biotechnology was granted support in the I edition of funding for student research and in the II edition of funding for Project-Based Learning under the Excellence Initiative - Research University program, by Rector's of the Silesian University of Technology Regulation No. 54/2020 and 55/2020 issued March 13, 2020, and grants 02/040/BK_20/0002 (Magdalena Skonieczna and Dorota Hudy), and 02/040/BKM_20/0005 (Małgorzata Adamiec).

References

1. Dukes, C.E.: The classification of cancer of the rectum. J. Pathol. **35**, 323–332 (1932)
2. Matsuyama, Y., Takao, S., Aikou, T.: Comparison of matrix metalloproteinase expression between primary tumors with or without liver metastasis in pancreatic and colorectal carcinomas. J. Surg. Oncol. **80**(2), 105–110 (2002)
3. Li, B.H., Zhao, P., Liu, S.Z., Yu, Y.M., Han, M., Wen, J.K.: Matrix metalloproteinase-2 and tissue inhibitor of metalloproteinase-2 in colorectal carcinoma invasion and metastasis. World J. Gastroenterol. **11**, 3046–50 (2005)
4. Korbicz, J., Maniewski, R., Patan, K., Kowal, M. (eds.); Current trends in biomedical engineering and bioimages analysis. In: Proceedings of the 21st Polish Conference on Biocybernetics and Biomedical Engineering (PCBEE 2019). AISC, vol. 1033. Springer, Cham (2020). https://doi.org/10.1007/978-3-030-29885-2
5. Skonieczna, M., Hudy, D., Hejmo, T., Buldak, R.J., Adamiec, M., Kukla, M.: The adipokine vaspin reduces apoptosis in human hepatocellular carcinoma (Hep-3B) cells, associated with lower levels of NO and superoxide anion. BMC Pharmacol. Toxicol. **20**, 58 (2019)
6. Skonieczna, M., Adamiec, M., Hudy, D., Niesłoń, P., Fochtman, D., Bil, P.: Live impedance measurements and time-lapse microscopy observations of cellular adhesion, proliferation and migration after ionizing radiation. Curr. Pharm. Biotechnol. **21**(7), 642–652 (2020)
7. Ehrig, K., Kilinc, M.O., Chen, N.G., et al.: Growth inhibition of different human colorectal cancer xenografts after a single intravenous injection of oncolytic vaccinia virus GLV-1h68. J Transl Med **11**, 79 (2013)
8. Yusof, H.M., Ab-Rahim, S., Wan Ngah, W.Z., Nathan, S., Jamal, A.R.A., Mazlan, M.: Metabolites profile of colorectal cancer cells at different stages. Int. J. Appl. Pharm. **11**(5), 66–70 (2019)

9. Shabahang, M., Buras, R.R., Davoodi, F., Schumaker, L.M., Nauta, R.J., Evans, S.R.T.: 1,25-Dihydroxyvitamin D3 receptor as a marker of human colon carcinoma cell line differentiation and growth inhibition, Cancer Res. **53**, 3712–3718 (1993)
10. Ferenac, M., Polančec, D., Huzak, M., Pereira-Smith, O.M., Rubelj, I.: Early-senescing human skin fibroblasts do not demonstrate accelerated telomere shortening. J. Gerontol. Ser. A **60**(7), 820–829 (2005)
11. Gupta, A., Mugundu, G.M., Desai, P.B., Thummel, K.E., Unadkat, J.D.: Intestinal human colon adenocarcinoma cell line LS180 is an excellent model to study pregnane X receptor, but not constitutive androstane receptor, mediated CYP3A4 and multidrug resistance transporter 1 induction: studies with anti-human immunodeficiency virus protease inhibitors. Drug Metab. Dispos. **36**(6), 1172–80 (2008)
12. Bułdak, R.J., et al.: Changes in subcellular localization of visfatin in human colorectal HCT-116 carcinoma cell line after cytochalasin B treatment. Eur. J. Histochem. **58**(3), 2408 (2014)
13. Buldak, R.J., et al.: Exogenous administration of visfatin affects cytokine secretion and increases oxidative stress in human malignant melanoma Me45 cells. J. Physiol. Pharmacol. **64**(3), 377–385 (2013)
14. Douglas, H., Robert, A.: Weinberg Cell, vol. 100, pp. 57–70, Cell Press (2000)
15. Douglas, H., Robert, A.: Weinberg Cell, vol. 144, Elsevier Inc., New York (2011)

An Alternative Methodology for Preparation of Bacterial Samples for Stratospheric Balloon Flight: Comparison Between High Density Wet Pellet and Medium Density Glycerol Solution

Ignacy Górecki[1(✉)], Arkadiusz Kołodziej[1], Agata Kołodziejczyk[2], Matt Harasymczuk[2], and Ksenia Szymanek-Majchrzak[3]

[1] Students' Scientific Group, Chair and Department of Medical Microbiology, Medical University of Warsaw, Warsaw, Poland
s074444@student.wum.edu.pl

[2] Analog Astronaut Training Center, Cracow, Poland

[3] Chair and Department of Medical Microbiology, Medical University of Warsaw, Warsaw, Poland

Abstract. Introduction: Micro-aerosols containing bacteria can be found in extreme conditions of the terrestrial stratosphere. Lyophilization is a standard method for preparing bacterial samples for stratospheric balloon flights. Here we compare the viability of bacteria prepared according to different methods: high- density wet pellets and medium-density broth suspension with glycerol before and after a stratospheric balloon flight in order to establish an effective and accessible method alternative to lyophilization.

Methods: Subjects of our study were bacteria causing hospital-acquired infections. One set of samples was prepared as a wet pellet. The second set of samples was obtained by adding brain heart infusion broth with 15% glycerol solution to the wet pellets. Each set had an additional group with protective layer of aluminum foil. A viable count assay was performed by preparing series of dilutions and calculating Colony Forming Units (CFU/ml). Next, we compared the data between two sets before and after a single stratospheric flight.

Results: Majority of the bacterial strains (72,8%) showed a higher survival rate suspended in a glycerol solution. Carbapenem-resistant *E. coli* pellet samples had higher viability. Results for *P. aeruginosa* were inconclusive, because CFU numbers varied between different sets and groups. Therefore, no obvious trend in survival could be observed.

Conclusions: Although lyophilization of bacterial samples may still be the most popular method, it is not necessarily required to perform basic stratospheric balloon flight experiments. Both our methods used with this set of bacteria allow most of them to survive a stratospheric balloon flight, however the glycerol supplement seems to give better protection. It is possible that different species require different approach.

Keywords: Astrobiology · Bacterial sample · Glycerol solution · Stratospheric balloon flight · Wet pellet

N. Piaseczna et al. (Eds.): EMBS ICS 2020, AISC 1360, pp. 33–38, 2022.
https://doi.org/10.1007/978-3-030-88976-0_5

1 Introduction

Terrestrial stratosphere (ca. 12/18 - 50 km above sea level - ABL) is an area with extremely unfavorable conditions. However, studies have shown that alive bacteria can be isolated from the stratosphere in the form of micro-aerosols, which is of interest for researchers in fields such as astrobiology, microbiology or studies on Earth's atmosphere [1,2].

Only a fraction of microorganisms that get to higher atmospheres survive due to harsh conditions such as ultraviolet (UV) and cosmic (ionizing) radiation, ozone, temperature fluctuations, hypobaric pressure, desiccation, and starvation. Such factors have a great impact on organisms and can inhibit their growth and survival [2,3]. Stratospheric balloon flights are widely performed by researchers and organizations like NASA (National Aeronautics and Space Administration) [4].

Biological research requires keeping the organisms under investigation alive in order to perform analyses. To achieve that, bacterial samples have been usually prepared using lyophilization (freeze-drying), which is a low temperature dehydration process, that inhibits bacteria's metabolism [5]. Therefore, there is a need for an alternative and universal method that is accessible for every laboratory.

We aim to establish such method. Here we compare the viability of bacteria prepared as high-density wet pellets (HDWP) and medium density broth suspension with glycerol (MDGS) before and after a stratospheric balloon flight.

2 Materials and Methods

2.1 Bacterial Cultures

Model bacterial strains acquired from ATCC (American Type Culture Collection):

- *Escherichia coli* (ATCC 25922),
- *Klebsiella pneumoniae* (ATCC 700603),
- *Pseudomonas aeruginosa* (ATCC 27853),
- *Enterococcus faecalis* (ATCC 29212), and
- *Staphylococcus aureus* (ATCC 25923)

generally sensitive to antibiotics as well as:

- carbapenem resistant *E. coli* (CPE),
- carbapenem resistant *K. pneumoniae* (CPE),
- multi-drug resistant *P. aeruginosa* (MDR),
- vancomycin resistant *E. faecalis* (VRE),
- methicillin resistant/vancomycin sensitive *S. aureus* (MRSA/VSSA), and
- methicillin resistant/vancomycin intermediate *S. aureus* (MRSA/VISA)

were obtained from stocks owned by the Chair and Department of Medical Microbiology, Medical University of Warsaw.

2.2 Sample Preparation

44 aliquots of 1 ml of bacterial suspension of each strain with optical density 2,0 MacF were used to create high density wet pellets. Aliquots were divided into two sets (22 aliquots each):

1. I set - high density pellets were the final samples;
2. II set - to high density wet pellets 100 µl of brain heart infusion broth (BHI-B) medium with 15% glycerol solution was added obtaining medium density glycerol solution.

Before installing the samples on board the capsule of the stratospheric balloon, each set was divided into two groups (11 samples each): one without cover and the second with a covering layer of aluminum foil as an isolation from sunlight, UV radiation and temperature. Each group had the same set of bacterial strains.

2.3 Viable Count Assay

- Before flight: From the starting colonies 100 µl of bacterial suspension was used to prepare a series of dilutions (10^{-5}, 10^{-6}, 10^{-7}). Cultures on agar plates were used to calculate Colony Forming Units (CFU/ml),
- After flight: Samples from I set were resuspended in 100 µl of BHI-B medium. 50 µl of bacterial suspension from both sets were cultured on agar plates. For group without cover, dilutions 10^{-1}, 10^{-2}, 10^{-3} were used. For the group with covering layer, dilutions 10^{-3}, 10^{-4}, 10^{-5} were used. From each dilution, 100 µl was cultured on agar plates in order to calculate CFU/ml.

2.4 Stratospheric Balloon Flight

Stratospheric Balloon Flight was performed as a series of STRATOS missions organized by Analog Astronaut Training Center (www.astronaut.center) according to the standard procedure (see Appendix).

3 Results

Results are presented as a comparison of viability between groups after the stratospheric flight. Numbers (expressed as a percentage) are shown in Table 1.

The majority of the strains (72,7%) showed better survival rate when prepared as MDGS both in the group with and without a protective layer of aluminum foil. Samples of carbapenem resistant *E. coli* prepared as HDWP showed better viability in both groups. Survival of *P. aeruginosa* strains varied between groups. Protected samples had better survival as HDWP. In the unprotected group, the model strain showed better viability as a MDGS, whereas both samples of multidrug resistant strain did not survive the flight. As MDGS is used for freezing the samples in −80 °C, for storage, temperature seems to be a great limiting factor for bacteria survival during stratospheric balloon flights.

Table 1. Viability post-flight. Colors indicate lower (red)/higher (green) viability. *Numbers based on approximation

Strain	Viability (%)			
	Unprotected		Protected	
	Wet Pellet	Glycerol sol.	Wet Pellet	Glycerol sol.
E. coli	0↓	1,11↑	0,089↓	90,6↑
E. coli (CPE)	0,00076↑	0,00036↓	0,067↑	0,00043↓
K. pneumoniae	0,0022↓	2,24*↑	2,17↓	~100*↑
K. pneumoniae (CPE)	0,000071↓	2,36*↑	2,36↓	~100*↑
P. aeruginosa	0↓	0,000014↑	0,034↑	0,00025↓
P. aeruginosa (MDR)	0↓	0↓	0,0076↑	0,0021↓
E. faecalis	0,00056↓	5,71*↑	5,71*↓	~100*↑
E. faecalis (VRE)	0,0003↓	3,08*↑	3,08*↓	~100*↑
S. aureus	0,00052↓	2,41*↑	2,41*↓	~100*↑
S. aureus (MRSA/VSSA)	0,0044↓	2,11*↑	2,11*↓	~100*↑
S. aureus (MRSA/VISA)	0,000026↓	3,45↑	5,26*↓	56,84↑

4 Conclusion

Although lyophilization of bacterial samples may still be the most popular method, it is not necessarily required to perform basic stratospheric balloon flight experiments. Both our methods used on this set of bacteria provide survival of most of them, however glycerol supplement seems to give better protection. It is possible that different species require a different approach.

Acknowledgement. This work was supported by a mini-grant from Medical University of Warsaw (project no.: 1M20/M/MG3/N/20).

Competing interests. The Authors declare that they have no competing interests.

A Appendix

The experimental mission was 2 h 29 min long and it was launched on 18th July 2020 at 10:30 CEST at Queen Jadwiga Astronomical Observatory in Poland, geographical coordinates: 49.7761 latitude, and 21.0901 longitude. 4 m^3 of hydrogen gas (Linde) was inflated into the 1600 g latex balloon. Scientific payload weighting 2 kg (with two cameras onboard and one tracker and parachute), was attached to the balloon. The balloon flight occurred according to the planned time, because the flight predictions were correct. That means that the balloon landing was planned to be located in a safe area within the borders of Poland. Flight predictions have been made using predict.habhub.org software integrated with Google Maps, available on internet. The flight track is visualized on Fig. 1 and Fig. 2.

The balloon ascending time was 1 h 43 min, while descending was only 46 min. Average ascend velocity was 4,825 m/s. The balloon burst at 31 km altitude. Tracking system was provided by SPOT GEN3 satellite GPS messenger. This device was used for flight tracking using 100% satellite technology.

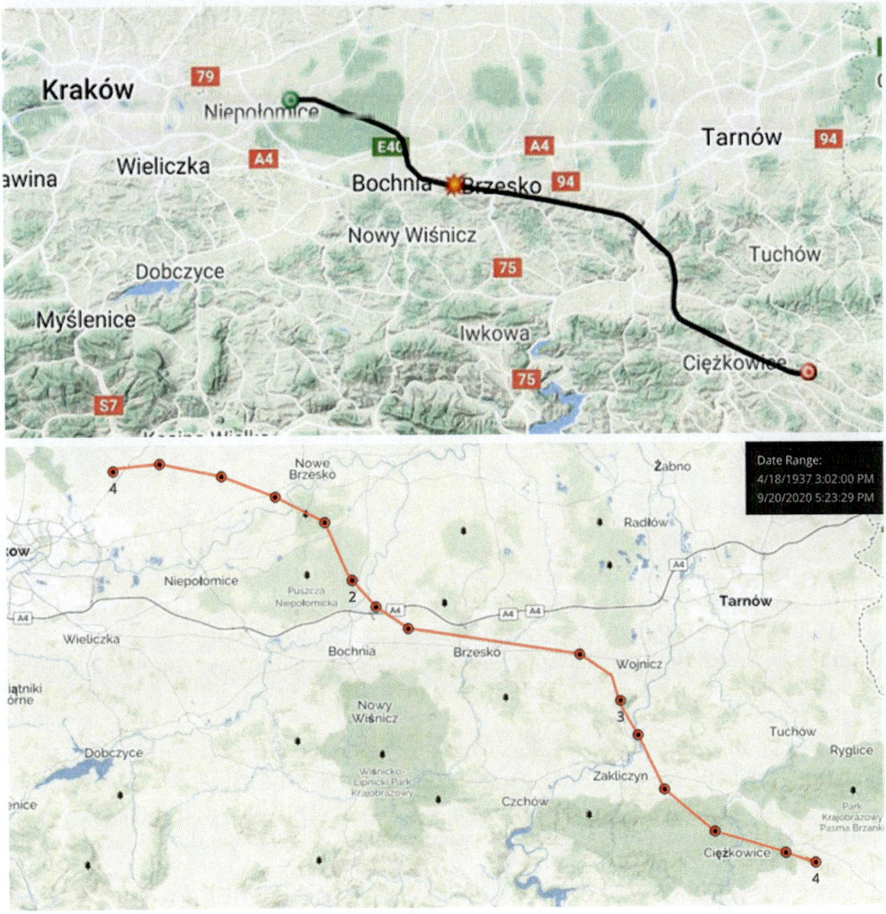

Fig. 1. Maps revealing the flight prediction and the flight tracking using SPOT GEN3 satellite tracking system during the STRATOS mission in 18th July 2020.

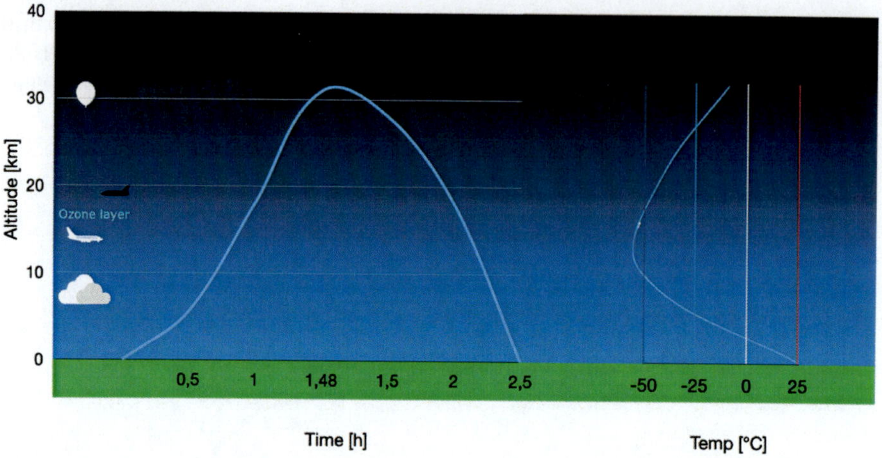

Fig. 2. STRATOS mission flight profile. The flight was 2.5 h long, with about 1 h exposition to high levels of UVA, UVB, UVC light. Balloon burst occurred in the stratosphere at about 31 km altitude. The graph on the right side visualizes temperature fluctuations at different altitudes. Curve was obtained as average from 4 temperature sensors located on the payload capsule.

References

1. Bryan, N.C., Christner, B.C., Guzik, T.G., Granger, D.J., Stewart, M.F.: Abundance and survival of microbial aerosols in the troposphere and stratosphere. ISME J. **13**(11), 2789–2799 (2019). https://doi.org/10.1038/s41396-019-0474-0
2. Smith, D.J.: Microbes in the upper atmosphere and unique opportunities for astrobiology research. Astrobiology **13**(10), 981–990 (2013). https://doi.org/10.1089/ast.2013.1074
3. DasSarma, P., DasSarma, S.: Survival of microbes in earth's stratosphere. Curr. Opin. Microbiol. **43**, 24–30 (2018). https://doi.org/10.1016/j.mib.2017.11.002
4. Khodadad, C.L., et al.: Stratosphere conditions inactivate bacterial endospores from a mars spacecraft assembly facility. Astrobiology **17**(4), 337–350 (2017). https://doi.org/10.1089/ast.2016.1549
5. Fonseca, F., Cenard, S., Passot, S.: Freeze-drying of lactic acid bacteria. Methods Mol. Biol. **1257**, 477–488 (2015). https://doi.org/10.1007/978-1-4939-2193-5_24

Comparative Analysis of Vocal Folds Vibrations Before and After Voice Load

Justyna Kałuża(✉), Paweł Strumiłło, and Paweł Poryzała

Institute of Electronics, Lodz University of Technology, Wolczanska 211/215, 93-005 Lodz, Poland
justyna.sujecka@dokt.p.lodz.pl

Abstract. In this paper, we present the analysis of the signals recorded by a prototype system equipped with an inertial sensor and a microphone attached to the larynx. The aim of the study was to compare voice parameters before and after the voice load. The results show the correlation between experience in working with voice and the score of the voice handicap index survey, i.e. more experience indicates a higher score.

Keywords: Acoustic voice parameters · Voice load · Fundamental frequency · Jitter · Voice handicap index

1 Introduction

The voice has a significant impact on our social life, enabling us to communicate verbally, but it is also a primary working organ in many professions such as singers, teachers, and journalists. Thus, these groups of professions are far more prone to voice disorders. Moreover, those people are often not familiar with correct voice emission techniques and vocal hygiene recommendations. Consequently, temporary or permanent disorders occur, which can lead to pathologies and harm the speech organ. This study aimed to develop an algorithm, which allows to determine the parameters characterizing vocal folds vibrations and to compare them before and after a voice load.

The human voice is a psychoacoustic phenomenon and its disorders can be evaluated by monitoring key voice parameters such as fundamental frequency, amplitude, intensity, time duration, and timbre. There are many tools available for diagnosis. Firstly, the listening evaluation was conducted by a phoniatrist during an interview with the patient. They assess parameters such as voice character, hoarseness, breathing route, etc. One of the scales that can be applied is the GRBAS scale in which each letter means other features of the voice (G – grade of hoarseness, R – roughness, B – breathiness, A – asthenic, S – stained). Currently, questionnaires are regarded as equally valuable diagnostic tools as ambulatory examinations, i.e., phoniatric consultation, laryngostroboscopy, or acoustic analysis. According to the definition established by the World Health

N. Piaseczna et al. (Eds.): EMBS ICS 2020, AISC 1360, pp. 39–51, 2022.
https://doi.org/10.1007/978-3-030-88976-0_6

Organization (WHO), health is a state of complete physical, mental, and social well-being, and not only the complete absence of disease or disability [1]. Speech organ dysfunctions may affect communication disorders through limitations in modulation, height, and voice loss, which may have a negative impact on the social and professional life of the patient. The most traditional method used for evaluation of the speech organ is the laryngological examination in which a phoniatrist examines the oral and nasal cavity and the throat. Occasionally, there is a need to perform a more invasive examination such as videostroboscopy. Nowadays, it is important to use the Ambulatory Phonation Monitoring – APM [2]. First of all, it is a non-invasive examination and allows for a long-term collection of data during the day. This is a small device that can be carried in a handbag or a pocket. The APM is equipped with an accelerometer that measures vibrations of the vocal folds. The sensor is placed on the neck, near to the larynx. It allows to monitor the basic parameters of the voice and their change as a result of various patient's activities.

2 Materials and Methods

2.1 Participants

17 participants took part in the study, 7 of them working with voice regularly (students or singers from the University of Music in Lodz) and having knowledge about correct voice emission technique (marked as S plus participant no. e.g. S3) and the other 10 individuals belonging to the control group (marked as K plus participant no. e.g. K3). The subjects were examined before and after voice load. In each group, the vocal load was different. Among singers, it usually was a rehearsal ongoing from 40 min to 2 h and the breaks were just for changing of notes, whereas among the control group the examination was conducted before and after the workday. Recordings were made in classrooms or rooms where were not additional people and no other sound sources were present, as this could adversely affect the subsequent analysis. These were not specially soundproofed rooms with a low noise level.

2.2 Device

The tests were performed using a device (Fig. 1) which was built in the Institute of Electronics at the Lodz University of Technology [3]. It measures the acceleration coming from the vibrations of the vocal folds in three perpendicular axes (X, Y, Z) shown in Fig. 1.

The accelerometer records signals with a 10-bit resolution in the measurement range of 2 g for each of the three axes and the operating bandwidth is in the range of 0÷2.5 kHz. The sampling frequency is constant at a rate is 5376 samples per second. The data is saved on a micro SD card in .bin binary files.

The sensor registers the accelerations associated with the movement of the vocal folds, which vibrate only during the production of voiced sounds. In order

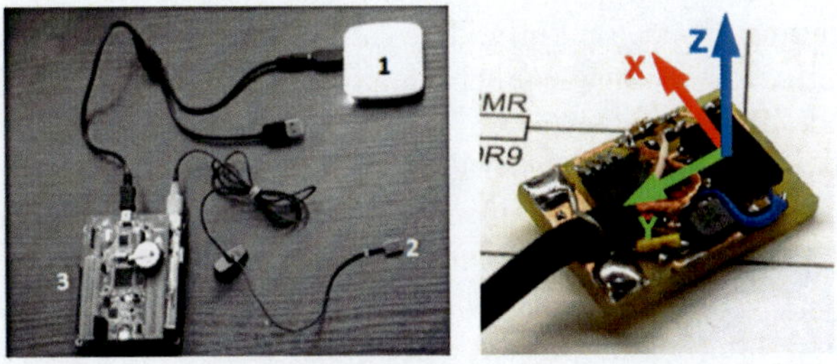

Fig. 1. The device used in the conducted experiment (left); layout of the acceleration axes of the inertial sensor (right). Source: Private source.

to take into account all directions of acceleration, the values of acceleration S(t) were determined, which is the root of the sum of the squares of accelerations along individual axes, i.e. x, y, z:

$$S(t) = \sqrt{x^2(t) + y^2(t) + z^2(t)} \tag{1}$$

During the examination, the accelerometer was attached to the neck, near the larynx with a medical paper patch. An example of the location of the sensor in one of the examined patients is shown in Fig. 2.

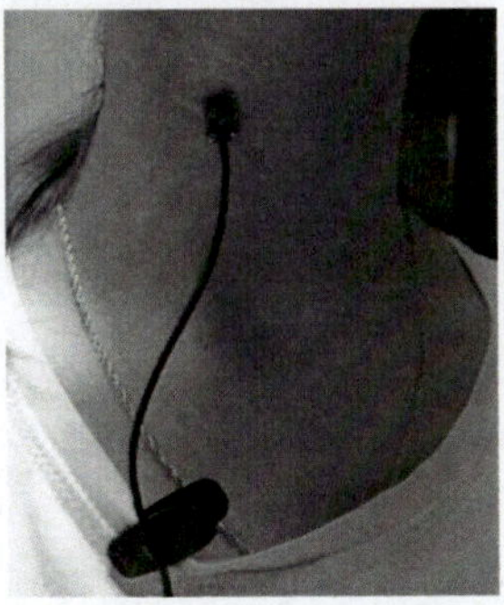

Fig. 2. An example of the location of the sensor Source: Private source.

The Cad microphone model U1 was used to record the speech signals. It is a dynamic microphone, powered by a USB connector, thanks to which, using a simple program for editing audio files, it is possible to make recordings directly.

During the test, the examined person was sitting on a chair, in a position that allowed air to flow freely through all anatomical elements of the vocal tract. The microphone was placed at a distance of about 20 cm from the face, but during the examination there were cases that the distance was changed. The examination has consisted of two stages performed before and after the vocal effort. The first was the phonation of the vowel "a" as long as possible. The second test consisted of reading a text for 1 min. The same fragment of the text was used for all measurements. Recordings from the microphone and from the inertial sensor were performed simultaneously.

All test participants filled in the Voice Handicap Index (VHI) questionnaire, which is an important patient's self-assessment questionnaire [1]. The questions are divided into 3 parts to evaluate the origin of voice disorders, i.e. 1) physical – appearing ailments, 2) emotional – the patient's feelings due to his or her voice, and 3) functional – impact on patient's life in the professional and social context. Each part contains 10 questions or descriptions of the situation. The evaluation is made on a five-point scale from 0 to 4, with the following annotation: 0 – never, 1 – almost never, 2 – sometimes, 3 – almost always, 4 – always. Points are counted in subgroups and then the total is added up. Individual score thresholds help to classify how severe is the voice dysfunction. The higher the number of points, the worse the patient's self-assessment of voice functioning. A total VHI score between 0–30 indicates slight voice disability; 31–60 – moderate disability, and 61–120 severe voice disability [4].

2.3 The Parselmouth Library

Additionally, the Parselmouth library (a Python library developed by Praat [5]) was used. This package allows to process audio files and perform their acoustic analysis. Parselmouth determines parameters such as shimmer, jitter, and average fundamental frequency. The library was used to compare the values of parameters determined by our algorithms and calculated by the Parselmouth library.

3 Algorithms

Acoustic analysis of the voice was carried out in two steps. The first is related to the processing of binary files containing signals recorded by the inertial sensor. The second step is the analysis of the signals collected via microphone. The following parameters were analyzed: the fundamental frequency, phonation time, shimmer, jitter, HNR (Harmonics-to-noise ratio), SNR (Signal-to-noise ratio), NHR (Noise-to-harmonics ratio), and signal power.

3.1 Fundamental Frequency

The voice is made up of many acoustic waves. The wave with the lowest frequency is called the fundamental frequency (F0) and corresponds to the vibration frequency of the vocal folds. This frequency has an impact on how the voice is heard. In the signal analysis procedure, the fundamental frequency can be determined in the time domain or in the frequency domain. The fundamental frequency was determined by two methods – the Fast Fourier Transform (FFT) and autocorrelation analysis with or without interpolation.

First, the Fourier spectrum of the speech signal was computed. The amplitude spectrum looks as shown in Fig. 3. Still in the middle part of the spectrum, for frequencies starting 1008 Hz, 336 Hz, there were harmonics of values higher than the other amplitudes for this frequency range. Due to the fact that a deviation may affect the quality of the analysis, the value of 0 was assigned to these spectral components. After processing of the amplitude spectrum, the maximum value of the amplitude was determined in a frequency range 0 Hz–2688 Hz. The fundamental frequency was calculated after the first 2 s of the signal duration and the minimum one second before its termination, so the voice should be stable, because usually in the initial phase there are larger vibrations of amplitudes and periods of F0.

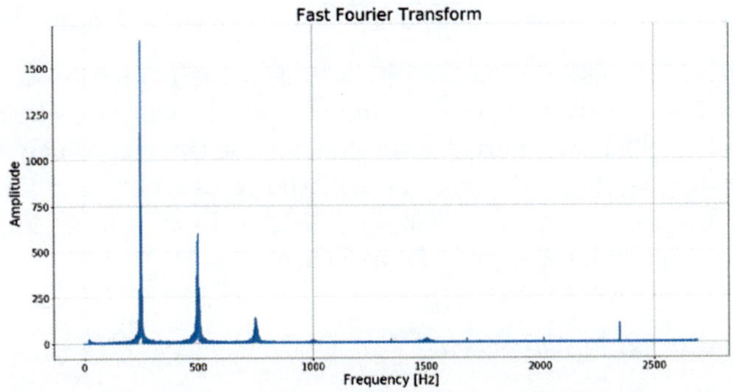

Fig. 3. Fourier amplitude spectrum of the speech signal. Source: Private source.

The fundamental frequency can also be determined in the time domain by determining the autocorrelation function. Similarly to the Fourier transform, the laryngeal tone was calculated for different signal lengths – 1, 5, and 10 s, respectively, and the selected signal fragment should be stationary. In Fig. 4, the recorded acceleration signal is plotted. It is necessary to determine the fundamental period of the oscillations in this signal.

The algorithm is based on the computation of the autocorrelation function of the signal. In the obtained function, we select the first non-zero lag maximum. Then we note the time coordinate of the maximum and denote it as our estimate T of the time interval of the vocal folds vibration cycle. Thus, the frequency sought is expressed by the formula shown below [6].

$$F_0 = \frac{1}{T} \tag{2}$$

3.2 Phonation Time

The phonation time was determined for both types of recordings (reading the text and phonation of vowel "a"). Maximum Phonation Time is the time of

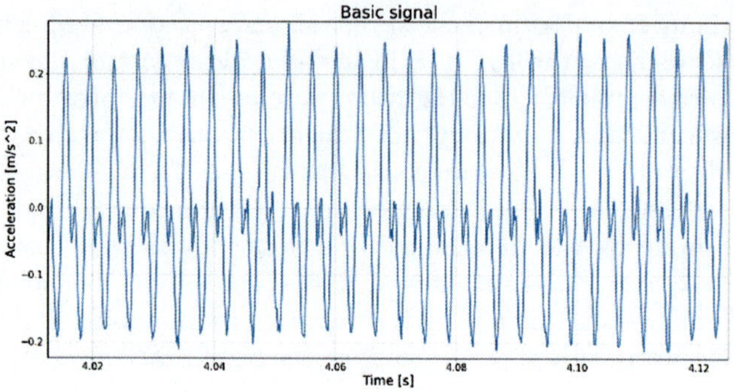

Fig. 4. Acceleration signal recorded by the device. Source: Private source.

effortless phonation period. The norm for continuous phonation is around 20 s. The goal of this algorithm was to eliminate all elements of silence from the signal duration, which was particularly difficult for the recordings in which the participants were reading. The variances of the results obtained for voiced and voiceless sounds were compared visually. On this basis, threshold values were defined, which determine the periods of silence.

3.3 Harmonic to Noise Ratio

The HNR is a measure that quantifies the amount of additive noise in the voice signal [7]. The additive noise is caused by a turbulent flow of air that is generated in the glottis during phonation. The HNR is expressed in decibels, a small index denotes asthenic voice and dysphonia, and a value below 7 dB is considered pathological. The following formula was used to calculate the HNR:

$$HNR = 10 \cdot log_{10} \frac{AC_V(T)}{AC_V(0) - AC_V(T)} \tag{3}$$

where $AC_V(0)$ is the detected maximum for the autocorrelation function, and $AC_V(T)$ are successive local maxima as a function of autocorrelation. The final result is the average of the HNR's calculated for each local maximum.

3.4 Noise to Harmonic Ratio

The NHR defines the ratio of the non-harmonic part of the signal (noise) in the range 1500 Hz to the harmonic part 1500 Hz, in other words, this quantity defines the noise content in the signal. The Fourier spectrum of the signal is used to calculate this parameter. Next, the index is found for which the frequency vector reaches values 1500 Hz and, according to it, half of the spectrum is divided into two parts – harmonic and non-harmonic. Then, the absolute values of the amplitudes are summed and the final result is the ratio of the sum of harmonics to non-harmonics.

3.5 Signal to Noise Ratio

SNR is expressed in decibels. This parameter is calculated by applying the Welch function from the SciPy package, which is used to determine the Power Spectral Density. A 20-s signal was recorded especially for this purpose, during which the sensor was not attached to the examined person and was stationary. The following formula was used to calculate the SNR:

$$SNR = 10 \cdot log_{10} \frac{P_{av}}{P_{noiseav}} \tag{4}$$

where P_{av} is the mean signal power and $P_{noiseav}$ is the mean power of a signal that contains noise only [8]. The same function was used to plot the power spectral density versus frequency.

3.6 Pitch Power

The pitch power was calculated on the basis of the signal amplitude of the constant time window width. The power was determined only for the voiced signal fragments. The power was then calculated using the formula below:

$$P = 20 \cdot log_{10} \frac{U}{U_{noiseav}} \tag{5}$$

where U is the sum of the squared amplitude values divided by the window duration, and $U_{noiseav}$ is the mean value of the minimum amplitudes from all silence windows [9]. Thus, the power was obtained for each phonation window. The final result is the average value of all phonation windows.

3.7 Jitter

Jitter is a parameter that allows to evaluate the relative changes of the fundamental frequency in consecutive vibration periods of the vocal folds. Jitter is defined as the sum of the differences of successive basic periods (Ti, Ti+1) divided by the number of periods (N) and is expressed by the formula [7]:

$$Jitter = \frac{1}{N-1} \cdot \sum_{i=1}^{N-1} |T_{i+1} - T_i| \tag{6}$$

Local jitter is expressed as the mean of the sum of the absolute values of the differences in consecutive F0 periods, divided by the mean duration of the base period. It is a percentage.

$$Jitt = \frac{Jitter}{\frac{1}{N} \cdot \sum_{i=1}^{N} T_i} \cdot 100[\%] \tag{7}$$

Jitter rap (Relative average perturbation) describes the relative change of the base periods with a smoothing factor of 3 periods (T_{i-1}, T_i, T_{i+1}).

$$RAP = \frac{\frac{1}{N-1} \cdot \sum_{i=1}^{N-1} |T_i - (\frac{1}{3}\sum_{n=i-1}^{i+1} T_n)|}{\frac{1}{N} \cdot \sum_{i=1}^{N} T_i} \cdot 100[\%] \quad (8)$$

Jitter ppq (Pitch Period Perturbation Quotient) defines the relative change of the base periods with a smoothing factor of 5 periods $(T_{i-2}, T_{i-1}, T_i, T_{i+1}, T_{i+2})$.

$$PPQ = \frac{\frac{1}{N-1} \cdot \sum_{i=2}^{N-2} |T_i - (\frac{1}{5}\sum_{n=i-2}^{i+2} T_n)|}{\frac{1}{N} \cdot \sum_{i=1}^{N} T_i} \cdot 100[\%] \quad (9)$$

Jitter ddp (Difference of Differences of Periods) is defined as the absolute mean difference between consecutive F0 period differences, divided by the mean base period [5].

$$DDP = \frac{\frac{1}{N-2} \cdot \sum_{i=2}^{N-1} |(T_{i+1} - T_i) - (T_i - T_{i-1})|}{\frac{1}{N} \cdot \sum_{i=1}^{N} T_i} \cdot 100[\%] \quad (10)$$

3.8 Shimmer

Shimmer is a parameter that describes time variations in the signal amplitude. Shimmer represents the mean absolute difference between the amplitudes for two consecutive periods (A_i, A_{i+1}), divided by the mean amplitude expressed as a percentage [7]. The quantity is given by the following formula:

$$Shimmer = \frac{\frac{1}{N-1} \cdot \sum_{i=1}^{N-1} |A_i - A_{i+1}|}{\frac{1}{N} \cdot \sum_{i=1}^{N} A_i} \cdot 100[\%] \quad (11)$$

Shimmer can also be expressed in decibels, then it is described by formula 12. It is the average absolute difference of decimal logarithms between two consecutive periods.

$$Shimmer\_dB = \frac{1}{N-1} \cdot \sum_{i=1}^{N-1} |20 \cdot \log\left(\frac{A_{i+1}}{A_i}\right)| \quad (12)$$

Shimmer apq (Amplitude Perturbation Quotient) is a relative change in amplitude with a constant smoothing factor of 3 or 5 consecutive periods. It is described by formulas 13 and 14.

$$APQ3 = \frac{\frac{1}{N-1} \cdot \sum_{i=1}^{N-1} |A_i - (\frac{1}{3}\sum_{n=1}^{i+1} A_n)|}{\frac{1}{N} \cdot \sum_{i=1}^{N} A_i} \cdot 100[\%] \quad (13)$$

$$APQ5 = \frac{\frac{1}{N-1} \cdot \sum_{i=2}^{N-2} |A_i - (\frac{1}{5}\sum_{n=2}^{i+2} A_n)|}{\frac{1}{N} \cdot \sum_{i=1}^{N} A_i} \cdot 100[\%] \quad (14)$$

The last parameter determined is the shimmer ddp, which is the mean absolute difference between successive differences between the amplitudes of successive periods [5]. It is expressed by the formula:

$$DDP = \frac{\frac{1}{N-1} \cdot \sum_{i=2}^{N-1} |(A_{i+1} - A_i) - (A_i - Ai - 1)|}{\frac{1}{N} \cdot \sum_{i=1}^{N} A_i} \cdot 100[\%] \qquad (15)$$

We applied the t-Student's test to verify if the differences between the parameters computed before and after voice load are statistically significant.

4 Results

The results of the conducted study reveal a correlation between the experience in working with voice and the score of the VHI survey, i.e., the more experience indicates a higher score, there is also a smaller scatter of the minimum and maximum values. Table 1 shows the average results of the VHI survey, divided into groups with different professional experience. The minimum and maximum values in each group are given in parentheses.

Table 1. Average VHI score in the different experience groups working with voice.

Experience in working with voice	Average result of the VHI survey
None	9.63 (2–39)
Up to 5 years	13.40 (4–37)
6–10 years	-
11–15 years	14.00 (8–20)
16–20 years	28.50 (24–33)

The largest sum of scores was recorded for the physical, then the emotional, and finally the functional part. This means that participants feel the most physical dysfunctions of their voice. The lowest sum of results occurs for the functional part, so it could be concluded that problems with voice do not disturb functioning in society and professional life.

We noted also that in the examined groups the vocal load alters the values of the phonation parameters. There was a relationship noted between voice fatigue and the laryngeal tone in the singing group, where the frequency increases. The results between reading and phonation of the sound "a" differed only by a few Hz, similar to the first method of determining the fundamental frequency F0. After the voice load, the fundamental frequency increased for singers at the average of 23.5 Hz. The noticeable increase after the voice load was also for the FFT method. Figure 5 shows the results of the fundamental frequency determined by the autocorrelation method without and with interpolation for the singing group.

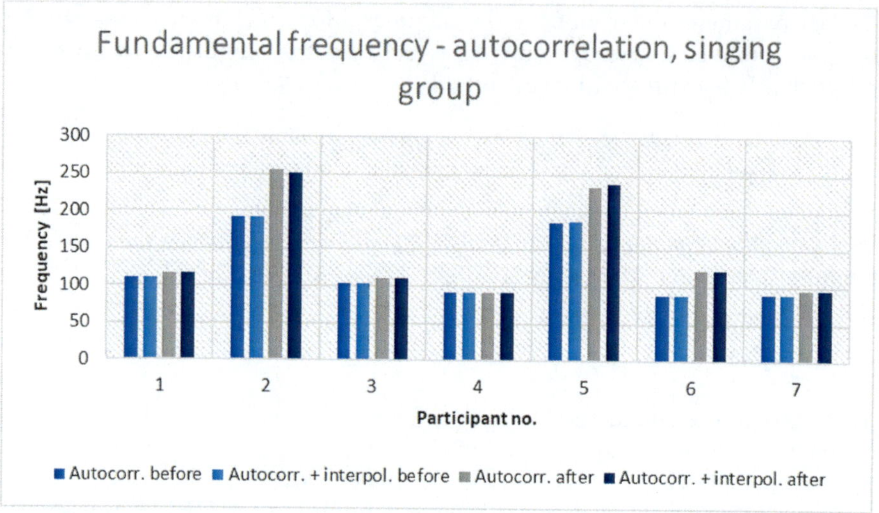

Fig. 5. Fundamental frequency, determined by the method of autocorrelation with or without interpolation, for the singing group and for signal duration of 1 s. Source: Private source.

The obtained results for the autocorrelation function differ from each other up to a few Hz when using interpolation. Thus, the use of interpolation does not improve the quality of the analysis.

Parameters HNR and SNR (determined for the phonation of the vowel "a"), decreased in five out of seven examined individuals in the singing group. However, in the control group, a decrease was noted in six individuals and an increase in the parameter values in four individuals. There was also no relationship between the pitch power and the voice load in both groups. The results of the NHR parameter are similar to the HNR in the control group – for six individuals the parameter decreased and for four individuals it increased. Similarly, in the singing group (for four individuals the parameter decreased, and for three individuals—increased).

The phonation time increased in six out of seven participants. That might be a result of "warming up" their speech organs. If the voice apparatus is more stimulated, it is easier to achieve such a prolonged phonation. There is no such association in the control group.

Among the singing group, the values of the shimmer decreased after voice load in five participants. Different results (increase) for S3 and S4 subjects might be due to a specific load. The voice during rock or metal singing must be loud and very strong, which significantly affects the load. Additionally, S4 individual is a teacher with many years of experience. In eight subjects, the percentage of shimmer increased after work. For the control group, the average increase in shimmer was approx. 0.05 dB.

Jitter is a measure of the volatility of the base periods. Among the singing group, the value of this percentage parameter decreases in five subjects. The

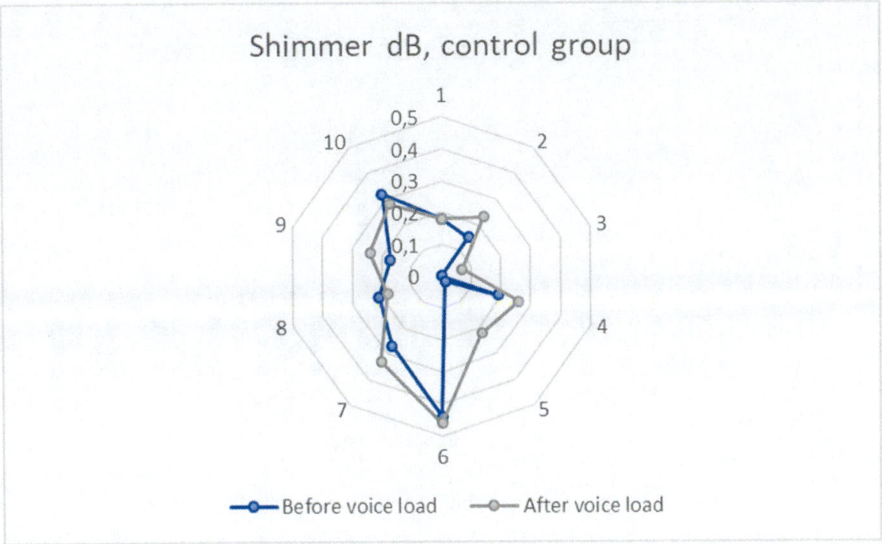

Fig. 6. The shimmer parameter expressed in decibels before and after the vocal effort, phonation "a", control group. Source: Private source.

same for the control group, the parameter values decrease in eight subjects after voice load. The percentage value of jitter (relative) decreased by 0.74% points among the control group.

It was planned to compare all parameters determined on the basis of the written algorithms with the results of parameters from the Parselmouth (Praat) package. However, the documentation does not describe the exact operation of the algorithms that are implemented in this package. The formulas are given but no information is provided on how the period F0 is determined. For this reason, it was decided to recognize the results obtained from our algorithms as the primary ones.

In the singing group, the probability of t-Student's tests was below 0.05 for the following parameters: fundamental frequencies determined by all methods for phonation of the vowel "a". Among the control group, the parameters with statistical significance are: jitter (relative, expressed as a percentage), jitter ppq5, shimmer (expressed as a percentage), shimmer (expressed in decibels), shimmer apq3, apq5 and ddp.

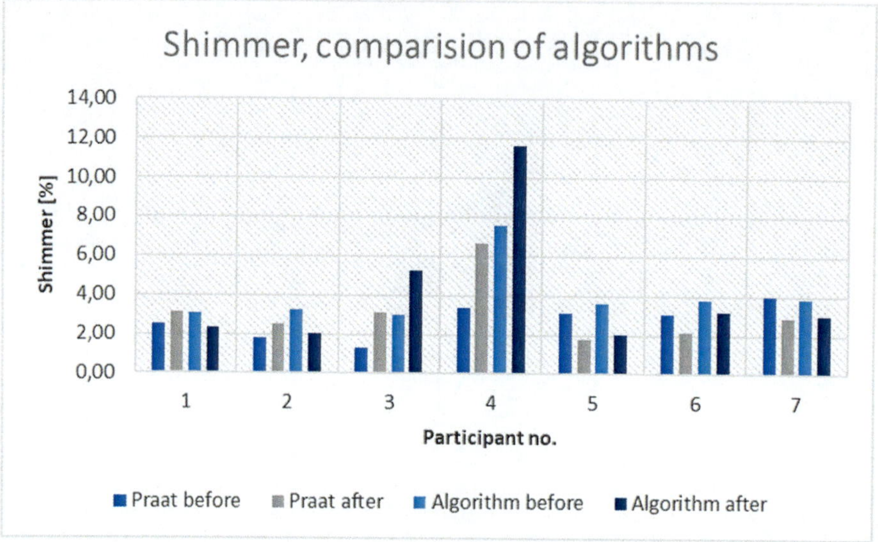

Fig. 7. Shimmer, results obtained from the Parselmouth library (Praat) and from our algorithms for the singing group. Source: Private source.

5 Conclusions

The study is an attempt to provide a quantitative characterisation of voice acoustic parameters before and after the voice load. The method reveals that the fundamental frequency significantly changes in the singing group of participants. However, it was the only parameter for which the statistical significance was proved in the group of singers, because the entire examination group was too small to draw general and validated conclusions. Despite the fact that among singers it was possible to notice trends in other examined voice parameters, the obtained p-value of the t-Student test exceeded 0.05 (e.g., decrease in the jitter value).

The method of determining the fundamental frequency does not affect the result. The differences between the autocorrelation function method and the Fast Fourier Trans-form are within the range of several Hz. Determination of the fundamental frequency is more accurate in the case of phonation of the vowel "a" than reading because it is close to a stationary signal.

The further direction of this research may be twofold. The first is to perform the test on a larger number of participants to increase the reliability of the research and allow for a more accurate demonstration of the influence of the voice load on the changes in the values of selected parameters, and to confirm it in statistical tests. The second option is to carry out tests in different groups of professionals to compare whether a given nature of the voice work may affect the tested parameters of the vocal folds vibration signal.

Acknowledgement. Authors wish to thank prof. Ewa Niebudek-Bogusz from the Department of Otolaryngology, Head and Neck Oncology, Medical University of Lodz, Poland for medical consultations of the conducted study.

References

1. Kuzańska, A., Niebudek-Bogusz, E., Woźnicka, E., Kopczyńska, J., Śliwińska-Kowalska, M.: Comparison of VHI scores in teachers with voice disorders and the non-professional dys-phonic population. Medycyna Pracy, **60**(4), 283–288 (2009), Instytut Medycyny Pracy im. prof. J. Nofera . (in Polish)
2. Nacci, A., et al.: The use and role of the Ambulatory Phonation Monitor (APM) in voice assessment. Acta Oto-rhinolaryngol, **33**(1), 49–55, Pancini Editore Medicina (2013)
3. Poryzała, P., Strumiłło, P.: A prototype of a personal, longterm vocal load measuring device. Elektronika: konstrukcje, technologie, zastosowania, **56**(9), 47-50 (2015). (in Polish)
4. Jacobson, B.H., et al.: The Voice Handicap Index (VHI) Deployment and Validation. Am. J. Speech Lang. Path. **6**(1997)
5. Parselmouth – Praat in Python. https://bit.ly/2WxZXyL. Accessed: 12 May 2021
6. Convolution and correlation. https://bit.ly/2LhQp5J. Accessed 12 May 2021
7. Teixeira, J.P., Oliveira, C., Lopes, C.: Vocal acoustic analysis – Jitter, Shimmer and HNR Parameters. Procedia Technol. **9**, 1112–1122 (2013)
8. Kowalski J., Pęksiński J., Mikołajczak G.: Estimation of the SNR in a harmonic signal using exponential smoothing. TTS **12**, 834–835. Instytut Naukowo-Wydawniczy "TTS" Sp. z o.o (2015). (in Polish)
9. Zieliński, T.P.: Digital signal processing from theory to application. Wydawnictwo Ko-munikacji i Łączności, 22 (2007)

Analysis of the Relationship Between Intracranial Pressure Pulse Waveform and Outcome in Traumatic Brain Injury

Agnieszka Kazimierska[1](✉), Cyprian Mataczyński[1], Agnieszka Uryga[1], Małgorzata Burzyńska[2], Andrzej Rusiecki[1], and Magdalena Kasprowicz[1]

[1] Wroclaw University of Science and Technology, Wroclaw, Poland
agnieszka.kazimierska@pwr.edu.pl

[2] Wroclaw Medical University, Wroclaw, Poland

Abstract. Clinical management of traumatic brain injury (TBI) patients primarily relies on monitoring of mean intracranial pressure (ICP). However, the state of the craniospinal space is also reflected in the shape of the ICP signal over a single cardiac cycle, called ICP pulse waveform. In this study, we aimed to investigate the link between the occurrence of different types of ICP pulse waveforms and the outcome in TBI patients. A Residual Network model was trained to classify ICP pulses using 21390 waveforms divided by an expert researcher into four classes ranging from normal (type 1) to pathological (type 4) and used to obtain classification results for long-term recordings of 36 TBI patients. Patients with unfavorable outcomes exhibited a higher incidence of waveforms of types 3 and 4 (median [first–third quartile]: 32% [14–92%] vs. 9% [1–14%] for the favorable outcome group) and lower incidence of waveforms of types 1 and 2 (68% [8–86%] vs. 91% [86–99%]). More frequent occurrence of pathological waveforms in patients with unfavorable outcome suggests the potential of using automated classification of ICP pulse waveforms in the monitoring of TBI patients.

Keywords: Intracranial pressure · Traumatic brain injury · Neural networks

1 Introduction

In the clinical setting, management of traumatic brain injury (TBI) patients is commonly based on monitoring of mean intracranial pressure (ICP) as increases in mean ICP are associated with higher mortality and worse outcome [1]. Cerebrospinal compliance, i.e., the ability of the craniospinal space to buffer changes in volume that precede rises in ICP, is, however, reflected not only in the mean value but also the shape of the ICP signal. ICP pulse waveform morphology, which is the shape of the ICP signal over a single cardiac cycle, is believed to

N. Piaseczna et al. (Eds.): EMBS ICS 2020, AISC 1360, pp. 52–57, 2022.
https://doi.org/10.1007/978-3-030-88976-0_7

contain indirect information about brain compliance [2]. Under normal conditions, the waveform is characterized by three distinct peaks: P1, P2, and P3. As brain compliance decreases, the prominence of P2 increases while P1 and P3 gradually disappear. Eventually, the waveform becomes rounded or triangular.

It has been suggested that the analysis of ICP pulse waveforms may provide additional information on the state of the cerebrospinal space [3]. However, the methods developed so far for the task of morphological analysis of the ICP signal primarily rely on complex peak and notch detection algorithms [4–6] which limit their applicability to pathologically changed waveforms as well as their usefulness in the clinical setting. On the other hand, a study by Nucci et al. [7] proposed that ICP pulse waveforms can be classified based on the overall shape of the waveform without the need for peak identification. The authors used an artificial neural network to classify waveforms obtained from hydrocephalus patients undergoing infusion studies with a reported accuracy of 88.3% and showed that the classification results correlate with alterations in cerebrospinal fluid dynamics revealed by analysis of full infusion study recordings. We are not aware of any studies that applied this method in TBI patients. Therefore, in this work, we aimed to develop a deep learning model for morphological classification of ICP pulse waveforms and to investigate the relationship between different types of ICP pulse waveforms and outcome in TBI patients.

2 Materials and Methods

Long-term ICP recordings (median length: 120 [92–150] h) from 36 TBI patients treated at University Hospital in Wroclaw, Poland (Ethics Committee approval KB-624/2014) were analyzed retrospectively. All patients were diagnosed with mild TBI with comparable clinical condition (Glasgow Coma Scale score, median [first–third quartile]: 6 [4–8]). The patients were treated according to the American Brain Trauma Foundation guidelines [8]. ICP was measured using intraparenchymal sensors (Codman MicroSensor ICP Transducer, Codman & Shurtleff, Randolph, MA, USA) inserted into the frontal cortex. The signal was recorded using ICM+ software (Cambridge Enterprise Ltd, Cambridge, UK) with a sampling frequency 50–300 Hz. The patients' outcome was assessed with the Glasgow Outcome Scale as unfavorable (scores I–III, 20 patients) or favorable (scores IV–V, 16 patients) at three months from the onset.

The recordings were separated into individual pulse waveforms using a modified Scholkmann algorithm [9]. 21 390 pulse waveforms were randomly selected from full recordings and manually classified by an expert researcher into one of five morphological classes: 1 – normal, 2 – potentially pathological, 3 – likely pathological, 4 – pathological, A+E – artifacts and errors (Fig. 1). Classes 1–3 reflect the changes in the relative height, width, and visibility of characteristic peaks P1, P2, and P3. Class 4 is used to represent pathologically rounded waveforms with no identifiable peaks. While Nucci et al. [7] proposed only classes 1–4, the additional class A+E was introduced in this study to identify artifacts and measurement errors, such as distorted waveforms, sensor calibration signals, or incorrectly separated waveforms, during the classification stage. The patients were split into two non-overlapping groups in order to avoid the correlation between waveforms obtained from the same patient, with 14 578 waveforms in the training dataset and 6 812 waveforms in the validation dataset.

A Residual Neural Network (ResNet) [10] model was proposed for the classification task due to its ability to extract morphological features from the data. 1-D vector of ICP waveform samples resampled to 180 data points and normalized to the interval 0–1 was used as network input. The model was trained for 100 epochs with accuracy in the validation set logged at the end of every epoch and used to identify the best performing version.

Classification results in full long-term recordings were obtained using the trained model. Occurrence of different waveform types, calculated as the percentage of each waveform type in all non-artifactual pulses, was compared with the patients' outcome.

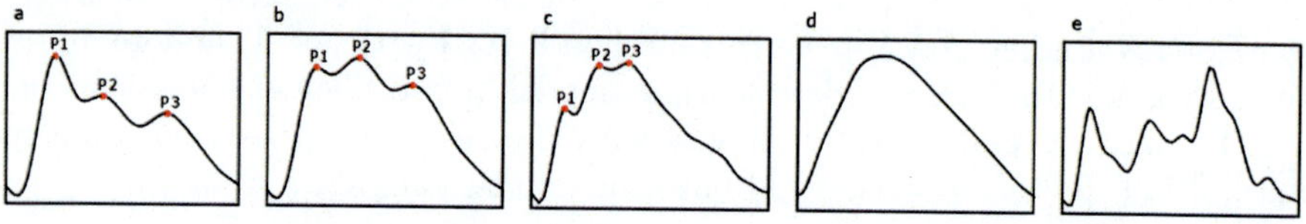

Fig. 1. Illustrative examples of ICP pulse waveform shapes in each class: a) 1 – normal: P1 dominates over P2 and P3, b) 2 – possibly pathological: P2 exceeds P1 and P3 but P3 does not exceed P1, c) 3 – likely pathological: P2 and P3 exceed P1, d) 4 – pathological: the waveform is rounded and the peaks are not identifiable, e) A+E – artifact/error: the waveform is significantly distorted.

3 Results

The model achieved a classification accuracy of 93% in the validation dataset. Detailed classification results in each waveform class are presented in Table 1.

Table 1. Classification results in each waveform class

Waveform type	Precision [%]	Recall [%]	F1-score [%]
1	99	95	97
2	92	93	92
3	87	90	88
4	93	89	91
A+E	77	98	86

Figure 2 shows the occurrence of different waveform types in data divided between patients with favorable and unfavorable outcomes. In the favorable outcome group, patients exhibited primarily waveforms of types 1 and 2 (median [first–third quartile]: 91% [86–99%] vs. 9% [1–14%] for types 3 and 4). Patients in the unfavorable outcome group exhibited an increased number of pathological waveforms of types 3 and 4 (32% [14–92%]) and decreased number of waveforms of types 1 and 2 (68% [8–86%]) compared to the favorable outcome group.

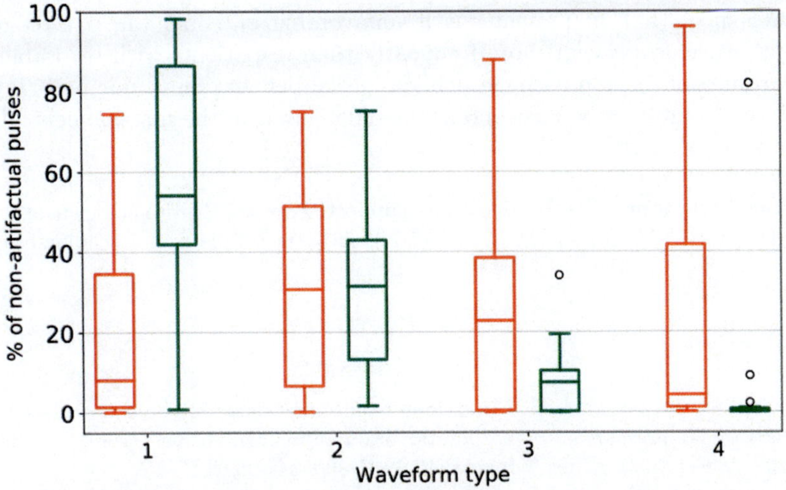

Fig. 2. Group-averaged occurrence of waveform types 1–4 in the unfavorable (red boxes, left hand side) and favorable (green boxes, right hand side) outcome group. Boxes indicate median (central line) and first-third quartile (edges), and whiskers extend to most extreme data points not including outliers marked by circle sign. (Color figure online)

4 Discussion

Despite previous studies suggesting the potential benefit of ICP pulse waveform analysis in patients with intracranial pathologies [3], this method is yet to be widely accepted in the clinical setting.

In this work we aimed to assess the possibility of using a deep learning model to classify ICP pulse waveforms obtained from TBI patients and to investigate the link between the occurrence of different waveform types and the patients' outcome. The ResNet model achieved relatively high classification accuracy of 93% in the validation dataset, with the lowest scores achieved in the arguably most varied artifact and error class. It has to be noted, however, that due to the preliminary nature of this study the model's performance was not tested in an independent set of data and manual classification was conducted by a single expert. The latter in particular may have influenced the results due to the operator's bias. Further study is therefore required to fully assess the model's generalization ability, including the introduction of a separate testing dataset, and the credibility of the results may be increased by providing manual annotations based on the consensus of a panel of experts.

Similarly, the incidence of different waveform types should be investigated in more detail to fully characterize how the shape of the ICP pulse is related to the patient's condition, since it has been previously reported that changes in ICP pulse waveform vary across patients as well as over time [11].

However, as classification results obtained from long-term recordings of TBI patients show that in patients with unfavorable outcome the pathologically changed waveforms occur more frequently than in patients with favorable outcome, results of this study suggest the potential benefit of introducing ICP pulse waveform monitoring as a secondary modality used in the management of TBI patients.

Acknowledgement. The research was supported by the National Science Centre, Poland (grant UMO-2019/35/B/ST7/00500). AU is a recipient of a scholarship from the Foundation for Polish Science.

References

1. Badri, S., et al.: Mortality and long-term functional outcome associated with intracranial pressure after traumatic brain injury. Intensive Care Med. **38**(11), 1800–1809 (2012). https://doi.org/10.1007/s00134-012-2655-4
2. Cardoso, E.R., Rowan, J.O., Galbraith, S.: Analysis of the cerebrospinal fluid pulse wave in intracranial pressure. J. Neurosurg. **59**(5), 817–821 (1983). https://doi.org/10.3171/jns.1983.59.5.0817
3. Heldt, T., Zoerle, T., Teichmann, D., Stocchetti, N.: Intracranial pressure and intracranial elastance monitoring in neurocritical care. Annu. Rev. Biomed. Eng. **21**, 523–549 (2019). https://doi.org/10.1146/annurev-bioeng-060418-052257
4. Hu, X., Xu, P., Scalzo, F., Vespa, P., Bergsneider, M.: Morphological clustering and analysis of continuous intracranial pressure. IEEE Trans. Biomed. Eng. **56**(3), 696–705 (2009). https://doi.org/10.1109/TBME.2008.2008636
5. Elixmann, I.M., Hansinger, J., Goffin, C., Antes, S., Radermacher, K., Leonhardt, S.: Single pulse analysis of intracranial pressure for a hydrocephalus implant. In: 2012 Annual International Conference of the IEEE Engineering in Medicine and Biology Society, San Diego, CA, pp. 3939–3942 (2012). https://doi.org/10.1109/EMBC.2012.6346828
6. Calisto, A., Galeano, M., Serrano, S., Calisto, A., Azzerboni, B.: A new approach for investigating intracranial pressure signal: filtering and morphological features extraction from continuous recording. IEEE Trans. Biomed. Eng. **60**(3), 830–837 (2013). https://doi.org/10.1109/TBME.2012.2191550
7. Nucci, C.G., et al.: Intracranial pressure wave morphological classification: automated analysis and clinical validation. Acta Neurochir. **158**(3), 581–588 (2016). https://doi.org/10.1007/s00701-015-2672-5
8. Carney, N., et al.: Guidelines for the management of severe traumatic brain injury. Neurosurgery **80**(1), 6–15 (2017). https://doi.org/10.1227/NEU.0000000000001432

9. Bishop, M., Ercole, A.: Multi-scale peak and trough detection optimised for periodic and quasi-periodic neuroscience data. Acta Neurochir. Suppl. **126**, 189–195 (2018). https://doi.org/10.1007/978-3-319-65798-1_39
10. He, K., Zhang, X., Ren, S., Sun, J.: Deep residual learning for image recognition. In: 2016 IEEE Conference on Computer Vision and Pattern Recognition, Las Vegas, NV, pp. 770–778 (2016). https://doi.org/10.1109/CVPR.2016.90
11. Ellis, T., McNames, J., Goldstein, B.: Residual pulse morphology visualization and analysis in pressure signals. In: 2005 IEEE Engineering in Medicine and Biology 27th Annual Conference, Shanghai, China, pp. 3966–3969 (2006). https://doi.org/10.1109/IEMBS.2005.1615330

Check for updates

An Algorithm for Matching Binary Airway Trees in 3D Images

Adrian Kucharski[1](✉) and Anna Fabijańska[2]

[1] Lodz University of Technology, 116 Zeromskiego Street, 90-924 Lodz, Poland
222486@edu.p.lodz.pl

[2] Institute of Applied Computer Science, Lodz University of Technology, 18/22 Stefanowskiego Street, 90-924 Lodz, Poland
anna.fabijanska@p.lodz.pl

Abstract. This paper considers the problem of airway tree matching in 3D images. An algorithm dedicated to chest scans of one patient obtained at different breathing stages is proposed. It assumes that the airway trees were already segmented from the 3D images. The method gradually transforms the moving tree to match a fixed tree, recursively rotating consecutive branches and their subbranches. The experiments were performed on 3D CT datasets of three patients, with images representing lungs in successive breathing stages. The assessment was made via the DICE coefficient between the fixed and the moving tree. Due to transformation, the coefficient increased by up to 30%. These results show that in the case of one patient, the proposed method can be an alternative to classical image registration approaches.

Keywords: Medical image processing · Airway tree · Tree matching

1 Introduction

Airway tree segmentation from CT chest scans is a challenging task. Due to insufficient CT scanner resolution and partial volume effect, some airway walls become discontinuous or partially invisible in the resulting images. As a result, region-based approaches to airway tree segmentation either leak into the surrounding lungs or generate reduced trees, i.e., containing only large airways, whose walls are usually continuous [1].

Airway tree segmentation becomes even more challenging in limited pulmonary opacification, which accompanies lung inflammation or acute respiratory distress syndrome (ARDS). In these conditions, some (even relatively large) airways become invisible in the CT chest scans, and the airway tree region becomes discontinuous. It is an additional hurdle for popular airway tree segmentation algorithms, which assume that a tree is a single connected component.

On the other hand, airway trees exhibit similar topology, which can be advantageous when the tree segmentation is considered. This is mostly in the case of the atlas-based methods [2]. These methods perform airway tree segmentation via

N. Piaseczna et al. (Eds.): EMBS ICS 2020, AISC 1360, pp. 58–64, 2022.
https://doi.org/10.1007/978-3-030-88976-0_8

registering the model of the tree into the input image. However, in the case of 3D volumes, image registration is a time-consuming and computationally heavy task, limiting the usability of atlas-based approaches in real-life scenarios. For these reasons, this paper proposes an algorithm of approximate airway-tree matching.

The proposed method requires the matched airway trees to be segmented. They should also represent one patient's airways at different breaching stages (see Fig. 2a). In such a case, the first (reference) airway tree is gradually reshaped to fit the second tree. The transformed reference tree can be next used to fine-tune the second tree segmentation accuracy. The method is beneficial when the airway tree needs to be segmented from one patient's limited opacity lungs during consecutive breathing stages, e.g., when monitoring lung aeration of the lungs in patients undergoing mechanical ventilation as considered by [3].

2 Algorithm Description

The proposed algorithm consists of several steps (see Fig. 1). The first one is to build the structure of the binary bronchial tree concerning its skeleton. Since branches are connected following a parent-children relationship, a data structure similar to a binary tree is used to model airway relations, with nodes representing airways and each parent airway having at most two sub-branches (children). The data structure encoding branch relations is next used when transforming the airway tree. Particularly, each branch with connected subbranches is rotated gradually by a selected range of angles. After each rotation, the Dice coefficient between the moving tree and a fixed tree is determined. For the final transform, we choose an angle that reaches the highest Dice coefficient. The procedure is repeated for every branch.

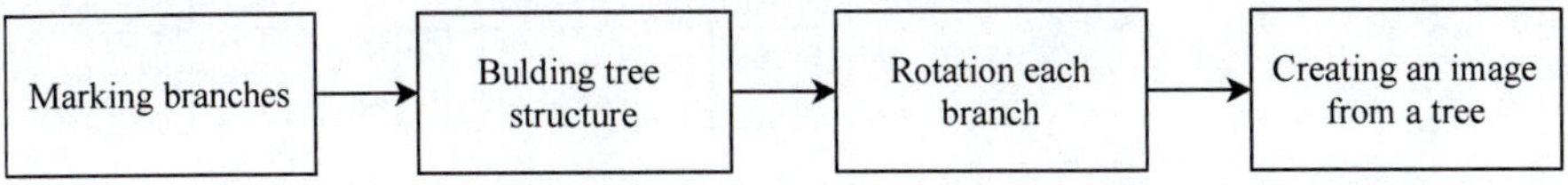

Fig. 1. The main steps of the proposed algorithm.

2.1 Labeling Each Branch in the Bronchial Tree

We first label each branch in the bronchial tree skeleton with a unique label to model the tree structure. To achieve this, we use an algorithm that travels down through the skeleton. To skeletonize a binary airway tree, we use the approach proposed in [4]. The starting point is the first voxel of the main branch skeleton (all other branches are connected to that one indirectly or directly). Based on the number of currently processed voxel neighbors in the skeleton, we decide whether it is a normal or a ramification voxel. Voxels that have two neighbors are normal ones and are labeled. Voxels with three (ramification) or one (last branch) neighbors indicate the current branch's end. They also indicate that we should assign a new label to the following voxels. We travel on the skeletonized bronchial tree using a stack (LIFO), to which we push not-labeled neighboring voxels of the currently processed voxel. Figure 2b shows a sample tree after executing the Algorithm 1 that details the above procedure.

Algorithm 1. The algorithm for tree branches labeling

```
U ← 1
Stack.push(start_voxel)
while Stack.is_empty() == False do
    V ← Stack.pop()
    if V.visited == False then
        V.visited = True
        V.value ← U
        if V.is_ramification() or V.end_of_branch() then
            U ← U + 1
        end if
        Stack.push(V.neighbors())
    end if
end while
```

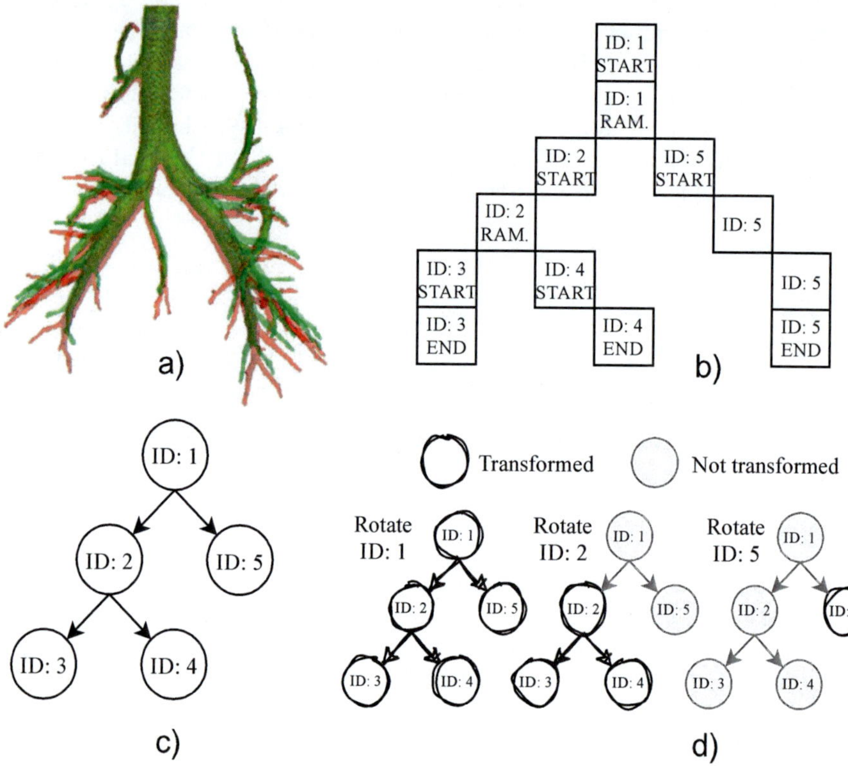

Fig. 2. Consecutive steps of the proposed procedure. a) bronchial trees in different expiration phases; b) labeling; c) modeling a tree; d) transforming a tree.

2.2 Tree Structure Modelling

The bronchial tree's labeled skeleton is next used to model the airway tree. Since branches are connected following the parent-children relationship [5,6], a data structure similar to a binary tree [7] is used, with nodes representing the airways and each parent airway having at most two sub-branches (children). Each node stores:

1. branch label;
2. an array of branch coordinates;
3. a left child (may be null);
4. a right child (may be null);
5. a starting voxel.

To find the above data for each node, we process each branch starting from the one with the lowest label. To find connected branches (children), we check which voxels are connected (directly adjacent) to the ramification. We calculate the Euclidean distance between voxels from the binary airway tree and the labeled skeleton to determine the airway tree voxels' coordinates assigned to a given branch. The assignment is made to the closest branch in terms of the Euclidean distance.

This operation is computationally expensive. Thus, to make the algorithm more efficient, we store each branch's coordinates and labels in the array. As a result, there is no need to iterate over the whole image each time. For the same reason, we store in an array coordinates of the voxels from the original image that we want to assign to their branches.

2.3 Recursive Transform of Tree Branches

The proposed algorithm's final step is transforming each branch and its sub-branches coordinates by a certain angle with a rotation matrix. We take the currently processed branch's starting position for it and its subbranches as the origin point. Due to the bronchial tree structure and its moves while respiration, we decided that it is sufficient to perform rotation concerning the X and Z axes. Important in this step is that when we process the current branch, we also transform its sub-branches, but we do not rotate its parent, so transforming the right main bronchus does not affect the left main bronchus. However, while we transform the primary bronchi, we also rotate the left and right bronchus. Figure 2d shows that, and Algorithm 2 describes the whole process. After transforming every full branch, we calculate the Dice coefficient between the whole transformed branch and the original image; then, we choose these angles which achieve the highest value of the Dice coefficient.

3 Data

The dataset contained five binary 3D images of the bronchial tree. The tree was segmented by region growing method [8] from the CT images of pigs' lungs. Each image had a size of $512 \times 512 \times 469$ pixels and contained a bronchial tree from the different phases of the expiration. The bronchial tree in Image 5 (im_5) was the smallest (i.e., had the lowest number of branches), while the tree in Image 1 (im_1) was the largest.

Algorithm 2. The Algorithm for transformation of each branch

```
function TRANSFORM(Node, z, x, origin)
    if Node not null then
        Rotate_Z(Node.voxels, z, origin)
        Rotate_X(Node.voxels, x, origin)
        Transform(Node.left, z, x, origin)
        Transform(Node.right, z, x, origin)
    end if
end function

Im ← Target_image
Root ← Tree_structure
Queue.enqueue(Root)
while Queue.is_empty() == False do
    Node ← Queue.denqueue()
    Queue.enqueue(Node.left, Node.right)
    D ← 0, X ← 0, Z ← 0
    for z in range(A, B, step) do
        for x in range(A, B, step) do
            N ← Node
            Transform(N, z, x, N.start)
            if D < Dice(N, Im) then
                D ← Dice(N, Im), X ← x, Z ← z
            end if
        end for
    end for
    Transform(Node, Z, X, Node.start)
end while
```

4 Results and Discussion

The proposed approach was assessed by means of the Dice coefficient measured between the fixed tree and the moving (transformed) tree. Resulting values of the Dice measure *before* and *after* transformation are presented in Table 1. Sample visual results are shown in Fig. 3.

The algorithm deals well with trees from comparable expiration phases. In such a case, after a transformation, we obtain the highest Dice coefficient (even above 0.9). However, for trees from distinct stages of inspiration or expiration, we can observe the lowest branches' deformation and tree matching with limited accuracy. Still, even in such a case, due to the transformation, the DICE coefficient increased by up to 30%.

The proposed method exhibits some limitations. Mainly, it is not always able to make a transformed tree to be a binary structure. Some branches may have up to three subbranches due to limited airway tree segmentation accuracy, insufficient resolution of the images, or noise in CT images. We should also take this into account while implementing the algorithm.

Table 1. The Dice coefficient before and after transform.

Fixed image	DICE	Transformed image				
		im_1	im_2	im_3	im_4	im_5
im_1	Before	–	0.841	0.720	0.625	0.552
	After	–	0.897	0.847	0.780	0.710
im_2	Before	0.841	–	0.817	0.697	0.608
	After	0.901	–	0.889	0.836	0.771
im_3	Before	0.720	0.817	–	0.803	0.685
	After	0.841	0.890	–	0.885	0.807
im_4	Before	0.625	0.697	0.803	–	0.782
	After	0.790	0.834	0.886	–	0.870
im_5	Before	0.552	0.608	0.685	0.782	–
	After	0.717	0.761	0.817	0.868	–

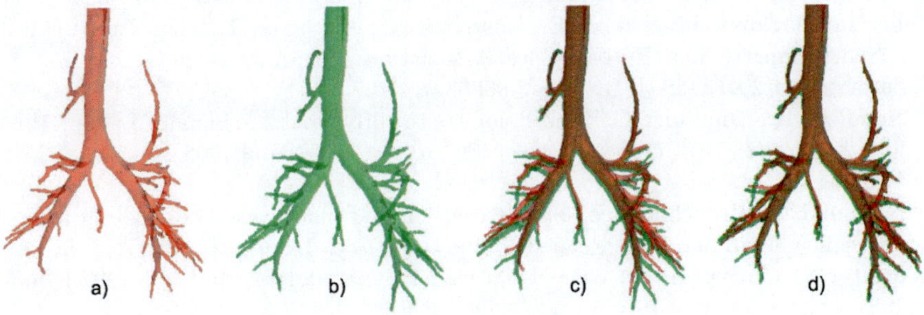

Fig. 3. The visual results of the transformation; a) the target image; b) the transforming image; c) overlaid images before transform; d) overlaid images after transform.

Implementation of the algorithm has not been optimized. A 3D CT volume processing lasts for approximately 110 s on the processor Intel Core i5-2510M. Additionally, the execution time depends on the image size, the number of branches.

5 Conclusion

Although the proposed airway tree matching method exhibits certain limitations, it can be an alternative for classical image registration methods. The main advantage of the approach is simplicity and processing time, which can be further improved via implementation optimization. This issue will be the next step of this work.

Acknowledgement. The authors would like to acknowledge Prof. Maciej Orkisz from University Claude Bernard Lyon 1 (CREATIS Lab), and Prof. Jean-Christophe Richard from Hospices Civils de Lyon for introduction into the subject of lung analysis in patients with ARDS and providing 3D CT lung images at different breathing stages used in this work.

References

1. Lo, P., et al.: Extraction of airways from CT (EXACT'09). IEEE Trans. Med. Imag. **31**(11), 2093–2107 (2012). https://doi.org/10.1109/TMI.2012.2209674
2. Iglesias, J.E., Sabuncu, M.R.: Multi-atlas segmentation of biomedical images: a survey. Med. Image Anal. **24**(1), 205–219 (2015). https://doi.org/10.1016/j.media.2015.06.012. ISSN 1361–8415
3. Pinzon, A.M., et al.: A tree-matching algorithm: application to airways in CT images of subjects with the acute respiratory distress syndrome. Med. Image Anal. **35**, 101–115 (2017). https://doi.org/10.1016/j.media.2016.06.020. ISSN 1361–8415
4. Post, T., et al.: Fast 3D thinning of medical image data based on local neighborhood lookups. In: Bertini, E., Elmqvist, N., Wischgoll, T. (eds.) EuroVis 2016 - Short Papers. The Eurographics Association (2016). https://doi.org/10.2312/eurovisshort.20161159. ISBN 978-3-03868-014-7
5. Horsfield, K., Cumming, G.: Morphology of the bronchial tree in man. J. Appl. Physiol. **24**(3), 373–383 (1968). https://doi.org/10.1152/jappl.1968.24.3.373. PMID: 5640724
6. Nakakuki, S.: Bronchial tree, lobular division and blood vessels of the pig lung. J. Veterinary Med. Sci. **56**(4), 685–689 (1994). https://doi.org/10.1292/jvms.56.685
7. Sleator, D., Tarjan, R.: A data structure for dynamic trees, pp. 114–122, January 1981. https://doi.org/10.1145/800076.802464
8. Justice, R.K., et al. (eds.) Medical image segmentation using 3D seeded region growing. In: Hanson, K.M. (ed.) Medical Imaging 1997: Image Processing. SPIE, April 1997. https://doi.org/10.1117/12.274179

The Stability of Textural Analysis Parameters in Relation to the Method of Marking Regions of Interest

Artur Leśniak[1(✉)], Adam Piórkowski[1], Paweł Kamiński[2], Małgorzata Król[3], Rafał Obuchowicz[4], and Elżbieta Pociask[1]

[1] Department of Biocybernetics and Biomedical Engineering, AGH University of Science and Technology, Cracow, Poland
arlesniak@student.agh.edu.pl, epociask@agh.edu.pl

[2] Małopolska Orthopedic and Rehabilitation Hospital, Modrzewiowa 22, 30-224 Cracow, Poland

[3] Faculty of Health Sciences, Jagiellonian University Medical College, ul. Michałowskiego 12, 31-126 Cracow, Poland

[4] Department of Diagnostic Imaging, Jagiellonian University Medical College, Kopernika 19, 31-501 Cracow, Poland

Abstract. This article presents research on the relationship between the method of marking regions of interest in radiographs and the stability of the textural analysis parameters of these images. 158 photos were collected from 34 patients of both sexes. The region of interest was marked in two ways on each photo and then analyzed using qMaZda software. Statistical analysis showed that parameters from the LBP group were very stable and that the results of GRLM parameters depend on the size of the ROI; also, GLCM parameters depend on the location of the ROI.

Keywords: Textural analysis · LBP · GRLM · GLCM · Stability

1 Introduction

The use of radiographs to analyze bone structure is a basic, significant element of medical diagnostics as they show all morphological bone changes, such as changes caused by demyelinating diseases that are related to inflammation, lytic states or age [1]. In addition to the shape of a bone and its density, which is distinguished by brightness in a radiograph, crucial information is also provided by the texture of the area. In the case of bones, their texture corresponds to their trabecular structure. The trabecular bone can be described with values such as volume fraction, thickness, or separation [2].

Interpreting a radiograph depends on the ability to assess it by the eye, which leaves a large margin of uncertainty, therefore it seems reasonable to use computer algorithms [3]. Known methods such as grey-level co-occurrence matrix

N. Piaseczna et al. (Eds.): EMBS ICS 2020, AISC 1360, pp. 65–74, 2022.
https://doi.org/10.1007/978-3-030-88976-0_9

(GLCM), grey-level run length matrix (GRLM), or local binary patterns (LBP) can be used to analyze such textures [4]. It is suspected that these textures could be dependent on the size of the region of interest and the composition of the bones, i.e. the cortical bone, the trabecular bone or the cancellous bone. The exact nature of these differences and their impact on the reliability of textural analysis is not yet fully understood. It seems natural to check the stability of the chosen parameters in relation to the method used to mark the region of interest, i.e., the shape and range of the region. The aim of this research was to assess these dependencies on the basis of orthopedic x-rays.

2 Materials and Methods

In this study, 158 radiographs of bones in the knee joint region were collected in the context of total knee arthroplasty (TKA). These images came from 34 patients who needed reoperations, mainly due to aseptic loosening (AL) of the implant, which is the most common complication and cause of surgery [5]. These radiographic images were obtained before and directly after these reoperations and during follow-up procedures. They were created using a Konica Minolta Regius CS3 X-ray machine and had a resolution (pixel spacing) of 0.175 mm × 0.175 mm. Some of the radiographs were made at the bedside and contain artifacts from various elements, including mattresses. The photo output format is 12-bit DICOM. During anonymization, the images were converted to the equivalent 8-bit PNG lossless compression format.

2.1 Region of Interest

Three regions of interest (ROI) were selected in order to estimate the textural characteristics of the bone: one at the tip of the prothesis stem (in the images obtained after surgery), and two under the tibial plate. One of the ROIs was on the lateral side and another was on the medial side of the tibia, adjacent to the cortex. ROIs were drawn manually by an experienced radiologist in two ways (Fig. 1): in the circular format (subsequently referred to as method 1), for which the average size of the selection was 3528.52 pixels; and in the precision format (method 2), for which the average size was 11966.02 pixels.

The precision format is more often used by radiologists because it covers the entire area that is of interest to the doctor; this format is usually chosen based on the radiologist's experience and should be located under the tibial plate at the tip of the prothesis stem, which helps assess the healing process after implantation. It does not have a defined size and shape, but what it consists of is crucial: it should show the trabecular bone without the cortical part of the bone and the periosteum. Due to its large size, it often contains artifacts or overlapping structures; therefore, such an ROI is selected according to the second method: a small circle in the middle of the structure of interest.

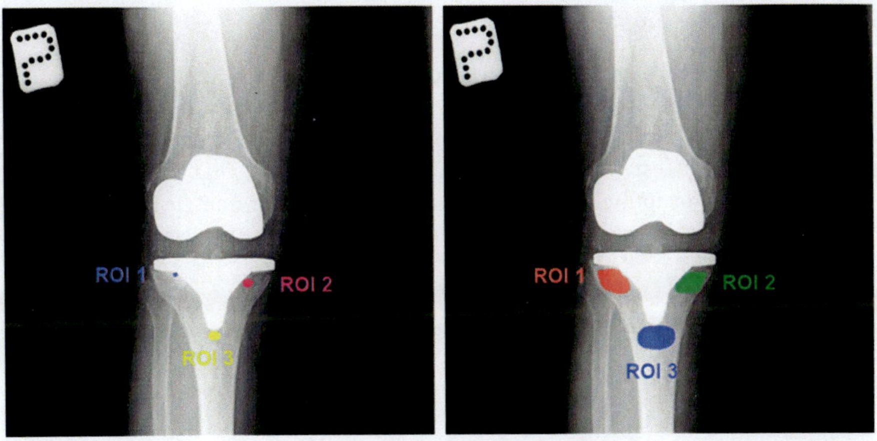

Fig. 1. Example of ROI marking in circular (left) and precise format (right).

2.2 Software

qMaZda software (release version 19.02, copyright 2013–2019 by Piotr M. Szczypiński) was used for textural analysis. It computes the shape, color, and texture descriptors of arbitrary regions of interest. Texture feature-extraction algorithms include the co-occurrence matrix, run-length matrix, autoregression model, brightness distribution statistics, local binary patterns, histogram of oriented gradients, and Haar and Gabor transforms [6,7]. Examples of the formulas for the functions used:

$$LBP(f_c) = \sum_{l=0}^{N_p-1} 2^i H(f_c - f_i), H(X) = \begin{cases} 1, x > 0 \\ 0, x \leq 0 \end{cases} \quad (1)$$

The above equation represents the LBP definition, where: f_c – midpoint, f_i – i-th neighbor of point f_c, N_p – number of included neighbors of point f_c [8,9].

On the other hand, the autoregression model can be described by the formula:

$$f_S(x,y) = \theta_1 f(x-1,y) + \theta_2 f(x-1,y-1) + \theta_3 f(x,y-1) + \theta_4 f(x+1,y-1) + \sigma \quad (2)$$

where the brightness of the image f_s for the coordinates (x, y) is estimated as a weighted sum of the brightness of four neighbors; θ represents weights, σ - error of f(x, y) value prediction.

The gradient magnitude map is computed according to the following formula:

$$|G(x,y)| = \sqrt{(I(x,y+1) - (I(x,y-1))^2 + (I(x+1,y)) - (I(x-1,y))^2} \quad (3)$$

where I is an image and x, y are pixel coordinates.

The histogram parameters (HIST) describe the characteristics of the histogram of the region of interest. The image brightness histogram of the region of interest or the neighborhood is normalized (divided by the number of pixels). In turn, the Gabor transform (GAB) locally decomposes an image signal to its frequency components.

2.3 Textural Analysis

In the first step, 3-sigma normalization was performed on all results from qMaZda. Then, the ROI size for both selection methods was compared. The value-distribution plot (Fig. 2) shows the significant differences between the data. The Shapiro Wilk test was also performed, which showed that in both cases the data were not normally distributed, while the non-parametric Wilcoxon test confirmed the statistically significant difference between the two ROI-marking methods (Table 1).

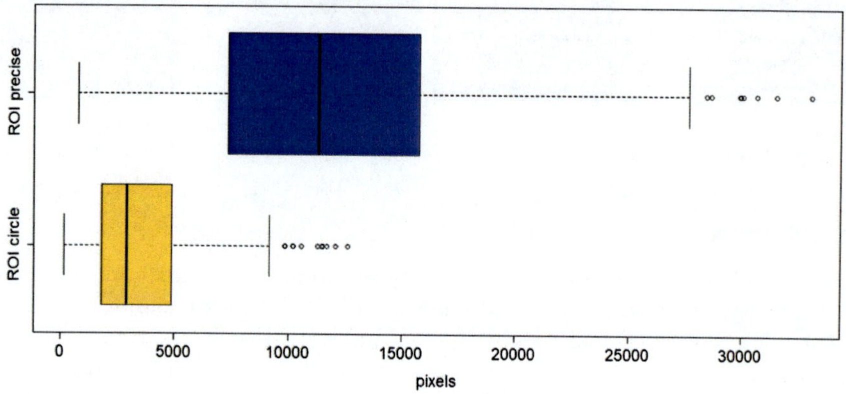

Fig. 2. ROI size distribution chart.

Table 1. Statistical test results

	p-values	
	Circle format	Precise format
Shapiro - Wilk	2.406e−14	1.221e−07
Wilcoxon	2.2e−16	

The next step was to calculate the Spearman's correlation coefficient between the parameters to show how much one ROI format depends on the other. In total, 293 parameters were evaluated with the correlation coefficient. For each ROI-marking method, Table 2 shows the mean correlations and the standard deviation of the parameter groups. It was immediately apparent that the number of images with ROI 3 marked was smaller than for the other two ROIs. This was due to the fact that ROI 3 was marked after the implantation procedure: the tip of the prothesis stem was clearly shown and its penetration depth in the bone was known. At baseline, before implantation, the size of the prosthesis stem is not always known (this depends on the condition of the bone and the prosthesis material). Therefore, ROI 3 is analyzed only after the procedure.

Analyzing Table 2 further, it can be seen that the parameters that are based on the autoregressive model (ARM) and LBP show high correlations in all three cases. However, the correlation parameters based on analysis of gradient maps (GRAD) or histograms of oriented gradients (HOG) differ depending on the ROI location.

Table 2. Mean correlations and standard deviation of the parameter groups for each ROI-marking method.

	n	HIST	σ_{HIST}	ARM	σ_{ARM}	GRAD	σ_{GRAD}	HOG	σ_{HOG}
ROI 1	152	0.204	0.108	0.604	0.178	0.315	0.204	0.386	0.062
ROI 2	152	0.250	0.160	0.734	0.093	0.449	0.215	0.602	0.069
ROI 3	111	0.385	0.159	0.775	0.100	0.596	0.120	0.725	0.030
	n	GRLM	σ_{GRLM}	GLCM	σ_{GLCM}	LBP	σ_{LBP}	GAB	σ_{GAB}
ROI 1	152	0.433	0.152	0.298	0.097	0.619	0.113	0.319	0.086
ROI 2	152	0.593	0.206	0.426	0.130	0.807	0.111	0.435	0.154
ROI 3	111	0.558	0.208	0.549	0.209	0.834	0.082	0.444	0.208

In order to better visualize the data from Table 2, scatterplots were generated. They represent all the parameters in each group of Table 2. The x-axis shows the values of the individual parameters for all ROIs selected with method 1; the y-axis shows the ROIs selected with method 2. The units on both axes represent the individual parameter values obtained for the ROI in a specific format. Sample LBP and GRLM charts are presented in Fig. 3; it can be seen that their angles of inclination differ. For the LBP chart, the parameters are tilted 45°. On the other hand, GRLM is visibly oriented more towards the y-axis, which suggests that the parameter values for ROI were overestimated in the precise format, which has a larger area.

Further analysis focused on three groups of parameters which, on the basis of the presented graphs and correlation results, indicated a common trend for all parameters, i.e., GRLM, LBP, and GLCM. A parameter was selected from each group for detailed analysis.

YS5GrlmHRLNonUni. This feature name consists of the GRLM stub to indicate the grey-level run-length matrix feature-extraction algorithm, followed by the letter H to indicate the direction of the runs. In turn, the RLNonUni function is expressed by the formula:

$$RLNonUni = \frac{1}{Area}\sum_{\forall l}\Big(\sum_{k=0}^{\theta} p(k,l)\Big)^2, Area = \sum_{k=0}^{\theta}\sum_{\forall l} p(k,l) \tag{4}$$

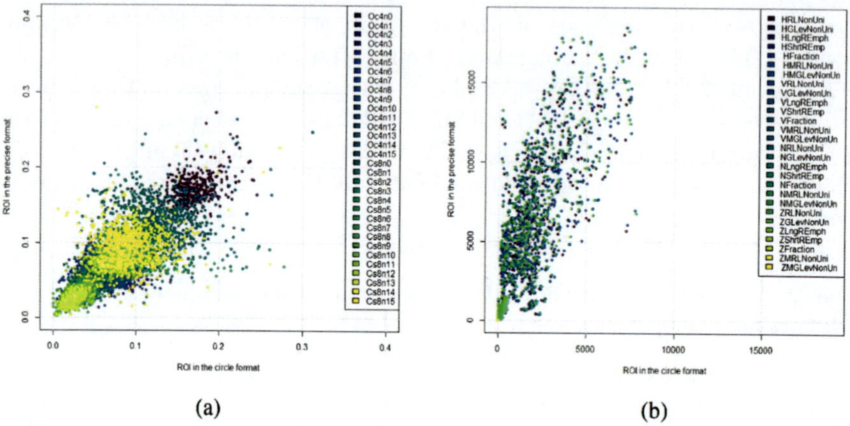

Fig. 3. Correlation graph of the parameters from the LBP (a), and GRLM (b) group for the two methods of ROI marking.

where $p(k, l)$ are counts of runs of pixels with the same grey level k and length l. Parameter $\theta = 2^n - 1$ represents the maximum grey level, where n is the number of bits per pixel.

The correlation of this parameter value between the two methods of selecting ROI was 0.673 for ROI 1, 0.870 for ROI 2, and 0.515 for ROI 3. To compare the parameter values obtained during the textural analysis and show the trend for each ROI, a Bland-Altman plot was created on which the regression line was marked (Fig. 4). The Bland-Altman chart shows the extent to which one measurement method differs from the other [10]. In this case, the methods of ROI marking are the compared methods. The x-axis shows the average of the compared ROI measurements; the y-axis is the difference between these measurements. The dark blue dotted line is the mean of the differences. When the line is not at 0, there is bias. In turn, the two light blue dashed lines represent the standard deviation between the differences. If 95% of the differences fall between these lines, then the differences are normally distributed.

The graph (Fig. 4) shows a significant bias towards negative values, i.e., the ROI selected with method 2 inflates the results relative to the ROI selected with method 1. On the other hand, a regression line showing a negative differences trend means that the larger the mean of the measurements, the more the values differ from each other. Therefore, it can be concluded (and this is also confirmed by additional graphs) that as the ROI size increases, the values of GRLM parameters also increase. The performed regression line coefficient test showed a significant result, thus confirming the significance of the trend and the dependence of the parameter on the ROI area.

YLbpCs8n2. The feature name consists of the LBP stub to indicate the local binary pattern algorithm, followed by Cs, which denotes the algorithm identifiers (center-symmetric), and then the number of neighbors, 8n. The correlation of

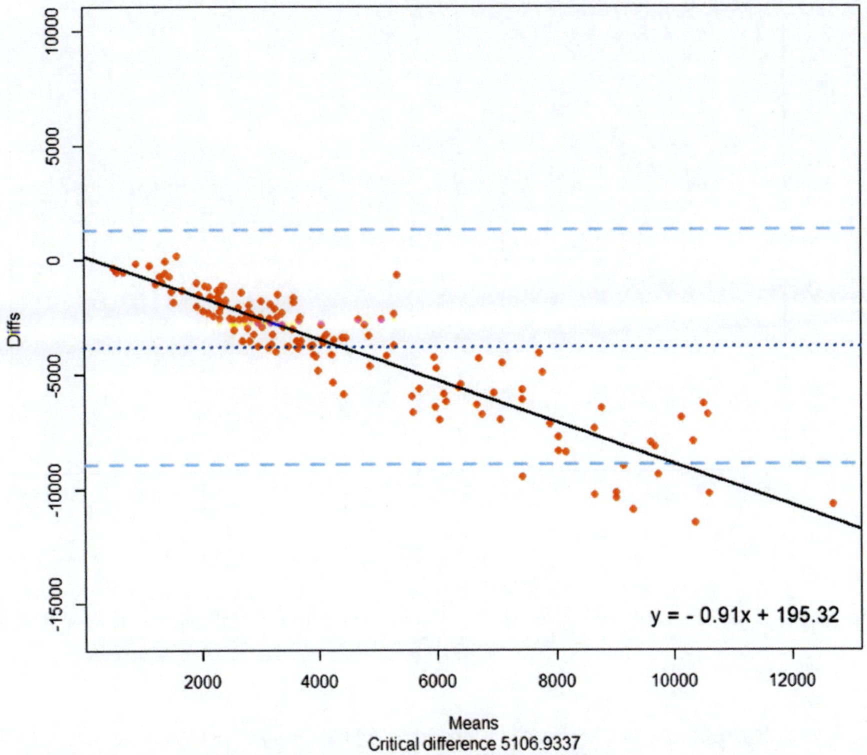

Fig. 4. Bland-Altman plot with regression line for the YS5GrlmHRLNonUni parameter for ROI 2.

this parameter value between the two ROI-selection methods was 0.734 for ROI 1, 0.886 for ROI 2, and 0.916 for ROI 3. As in the example above, a Bland-Altman plot was created to evaluate the behavior of this parameter (Fig. 5).

The chart above shows that the mean line of the difference between the measurements is practically at 0, which proves that both ROI-selection methods give similar results. Additionally, the regression line is not marked on the graph because it coincided with the mean line and its slope was not statistically significant, hence the conclusion that the LBP parameters do not depend on the size of the selected ROI.

YS5GlcmZ5SumAverg. The feature name stub for the grey-level co-occurrence matrix consists of GLCM, offset, direction and distance, and the name given by the above feature-extraction formulas. The direction is identified by Z. The distance is given by a number, d = 5. In turn, the SumAverg function is expressed by the formula:

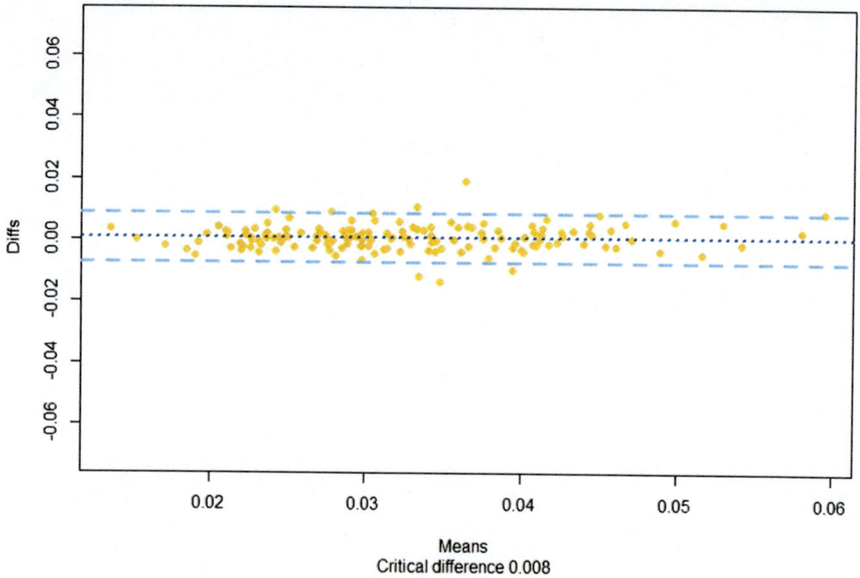

Fig. 5. Bland-Altman plot with regression line for the YLbpCs8n2 parameter for ROI 2.

$$SumAverg = \sum_{m=1}^{2^{n+1}} (mp_{sum}(m)), p_{sum}(m) = \sum_{k=0}^{2^{m-1}} p(k, m-k) \tag{5}$$

The correlation of this parameter value between the two ROI-selection methods was 0.151 for ROI 1, 0.254 for ROI 2, and 0.444 for ROI 3. The correlation is visibly lower than in the two cases analyzed above, which shows that the data is more dispersed. In this case, the generated Bland-Altman plots differ from each other: for ROI 3, the regression line (as in the case of LBP parameters) coincides with the mean difference line and its coefficient test has no significant value. On the other hand, a positive trend is visible for ROI, and the performed regression line coefficient test returned a significant result. Therefore, it can be concluded that the GLCM parameters are strongly related to the location of the ROI.

3 Discussion

The research showed that the most stable textural function turned out to be the one based on local binary patterns. Parameters from this group (including the analyzed *YLbpCs8n2*) had similar values, regardless of the type of ROI selected or its location.

On the other hand, the impact of the ROI-selection method can be seen in the GRLM and GLCM texture features. In the case of textural functions based on analysis of the grey-run length matrix, the size of the marked area showed a significant impact. The ROI selected with method 2, which on average was significantly larger than the ROI selected with method 1, was characterized by higher values of the GRLM parameters (this was shown by the analyzed *YS5GrlmHRLNonUni* parameter). In addition, it could be noticed that the greater the difference between the sizes of the compared ROIs, the greater the difference between the parameter values.

Parameters that were based on the analysis of GLCM algorithms showed dependence on where the ROI was selected. The analyzed YS5GlcmZ5SumAverg parameter showed that for three different ROIs within the same bone, the values significantly differed from each other. In areas where the tissue was homogeneous (e.g., the trabecular bone at the end of the prosthesis shaft), there was no noise or other disturbance: the parameters were stable and the values were similar for both small and large ROIs. In turn, in places where one bone often overlaps another (e.g., the tibia over the fibula), the marked area turned out to be significant. The ROI selected with method 1 more precisely marked the area of only the bone being analyzed, while the larger ROI selected with method 2 covered adjacent bones or other foreign structures.

This preliminary study shows that some parameters are related to the ROI-selection method. Conducting further studies will make it possible to determine the stability of the methods that are used in research on the prognosis of implant loosening in knee arthroplasty procedures.

Acknowledgement. This publication was funded by AGH University of Science and Technology, Faculty of Electrical Engineering, Automatics, Computer Science and Biomedical Engineering.

References

1. Dutra, V., Devlin, H., Susin, C.: Mandibular morphological changes in low bone mass edentulous females: evaluation of panoramic radiographs. Oral. Surg. Oral. Med. Oral. Pathol. Oral. Radiol. Endodontol. **102**, 663–668 (2006)
2. Tabor, Z., Latala, Z.: 3d gray-level histomorphometry of trabecular bone - a methodological review. Image Anal. Stereol. **33**(1), 1–12 (2014)
3. Borowska, M., Szarmach, J., Oczeretko, E.: Fractal texture analysis of the healing process after bone loss. In: Computerized Medical Imaging and Graphics, vol. 46, Part 2, pp. 191–196 (2015)
4. Strzelecki, M., Materka, A.: Tekstura obrazów biomedycznych: metody analizy komputerowej, pp. 25–38. PWN, Warszawa (2017)
5. Oftadeh, R., Perez-Viloria, M., Villa-Camacho, J.C., Vaziri, A., Nazarian, A.: Biomechanics and mechanobiology of trabecular bone: a review. J. Biomech. Eng. **137**(1), 0108021–01080215 (2015)
6. Szczypiński, P.M., Klepaczko, A., Kociołek, M.: QMaZda - software tools for image analysis and pattern recognition. In: 2017 Signal Processing: Algorithms, Architectures, Arrangements, and Applications (SPA), pp. 217–221 (2017)
7. Szczypiński, P.M., Strzelecki, M., Materka, A., Klepaczko, A.: MaZda - a software package for image texture analysis. Comput. Methods Programs Biomed. **94**, 66–76 (2009)

8. Ojala, T., Pietikainen, M., Harwood, D.: A comparative study of texture measures with classification based on feature distributions. Pattern Recogn. **29**(1), 51–59 (1996)
9. Smolka, B., Nurzynska, K.: Power LBP: a novel texture operator for smiling and neutral facial display classification. Procedia Comput. Sci. **51**, 15551564 (2015)
10. Bland, J.M., Altman, D.G.: Measuring agreement in method comparison studies. Stat. Methods Med. Res. **8**, 135–160 (1999)

Segmentation and Tracking of Tumor Vasculature Using Volumetric Multispectral Optoacoustic Tomography

Agnieszka Łach[1(✉)], Subhamoy Mandal[2,3(✉)], and Daniel Razansky[4]

[1] Faculty of Biomedical Engineering, Department of Biosensors and Processing of Biomedical Signals, Silesian University of Technology, Roosevelta 40, 41-808 Zabrze, Poland
agnieszka.lach@ieee.org

[2] Department of Electrical and Computer Engineering, Technical University of Munich, Munich, Germany

[3] Maxer Endoscopy GmbH, Tuttlingen, Germany
s.mandal@ieee.org

[4] Institute for Biomedical Engineering and Institute of Pharmacology and Toxicology, University of Zurich and ETH Zurich, Zurich, Switzerland

Abstract. Volumetric multispectral optoacoustic imaging has emerged as a new tool for visualizing the structure and the function of solid tumors in real-time. We aim to develop novel tools for 3D segmentation and tracking of underlying blood vessels to automate the characterization of tumors in vivo.

Keywords: Optoacoustic · Image processing · Volumetric imaging

1 Background

Volumetric multispectral optoacoustic tomography (v-MSOT) has enabled researchers to visualize not only the tumor anatomy but also study the activity of particular biomarkers and molecules. V-MSOT has opened up the possibility of investigating processes that influence the behavior of tumors in vivo at greater depths, with excellent spatial resolution and speed high enough to study perfusion profiles in real-time [1]. In the current work, we aim to use image analysis to segment vascular structures within solid tumor masses and track the perfusion profiles automatically. Previously, we have reported segmentation on whole body MSOT images (2D), in this work we extend them to segmentation of vessels and identification of perfusion parameters [2,3].

2 Method

The proposed 3D segmentation method consists of five main steps:

N. Piaseczna et al. (Eds.): EMBS ICS 2020, AISC 1360, pp. 75–78, 2022.
https://doi.org/10.1007/978-3-030-88976-0_10

1. wavelet denoising,
2. median filtering,
3. Frangi/Hessian filters,
4. binarization by adaptive thresholding,
5. morphological operations.

The flowchart presenting the whole process is in Fig. 1. First, 3D wavelet decomposition by Fejer-Korovkin wavelet was applied to the image, followed by 3D median filtering. The use of these filters was crucial to reduce the noise in v-MSOT images. The Frangi-vesselness filter uses the eigenvectors of the Hessian to compute the likeliness of an image region to be a vessel [4]. The Frangi filters are able to search for vessel-like structures with a specified dimension and compute the deviation from the blob-like structure within the mass. However, it is unable to distinguish between a line-like and a plate-like form of structures. In order to obtain a final binary volume mask, adaptive thresholding using local first-order statistics were employed. Morphological operations such as morphological opening and closing were applied to enhance the mask and fill the gaps. Finally, the identified blood vessels were clustered into different groups (3) based on the diameter.

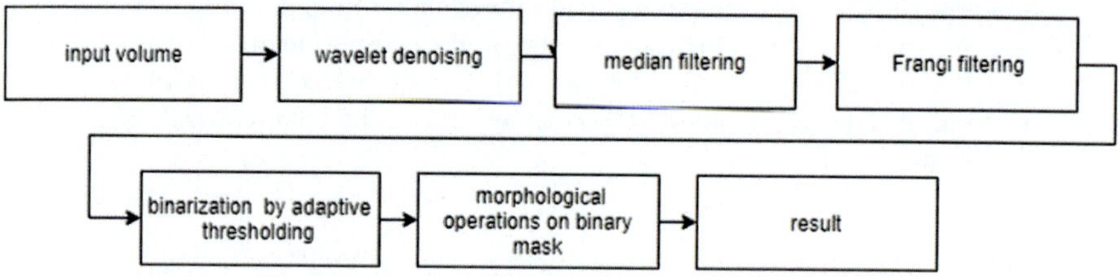

Fig. 1. The flowchart presents all five steps of the segmentation.

3 Dataset

The signal evolution was tracked over 1100 frames (20 Hz) to real dynamic and functional properties of the solid tumor mass. The imaged animals were five 8 weeks old female Hsd: Athymic Nude-Foxn1nu/nu mice, bearing 8–10 mm large tumour allografts. The tumours were grown upon subcutaneous injection of 1 million 4T1 murine breast cancer cells into the back of a mouse approximately 10 days before the experiment. The allografts reached a diameter of approximately 8 mm at the time of imaging. The imaging was conducted by custom-designed v-MSOT instrumentation with Indocyanine green (ICG) injections; animal handling was done under suitable approvals [5].

4 Results

In order to validate the segmentation method, five ground truth masks were created and the Sørensen-Dice coefficient metric was used, with an average score of 0.75 [3]. The segmented regions show a clear decrease of perfusion profiles, as supported by existing pre-clinical studies [1,5]. A slow clearing and extra-vascular deposition of the blood pool agent ICG can be clearly demarcated in Fig. 2.

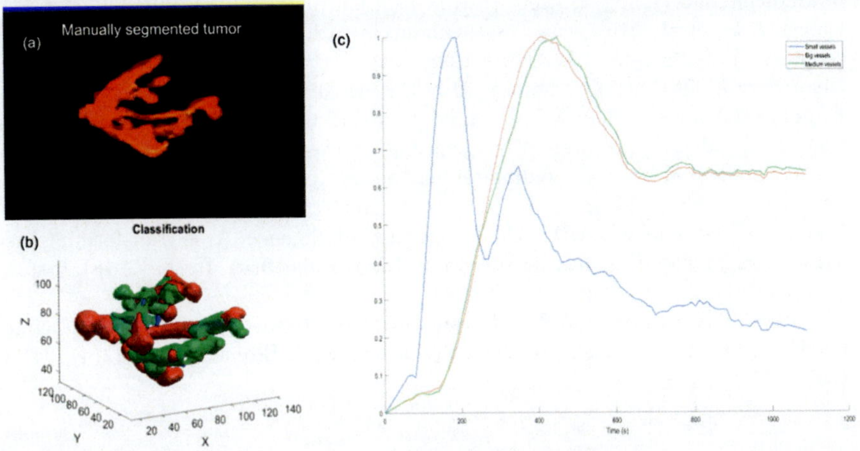

Fig. 2. The manually created mask (a), segmented vessels color-coded by diameter (b) – class 1 (red), class 2–3 (green-blue), and (c) perfusion tracking (1200 s) in different regions of interest.

The results are in agreement with the manual measurements carried out by 3 experienced MSOT imaging specialists.

5 Conclusions and Future Work

The proposed workflow automates the identification and clustering of blood vessels. ICG enhanced perfusion analysis reveals leaky vasculature, which is a hallmark of cancer. In our future work, we are extending the efficacy of the algorithms further, and integrating our solution with machine learning-based approaches [6]. We are hopeful that 3D segmentation methods will increase the clinical applicability, enhance the usability of MSOT, and encourage the translation of the v-MSOT technology to regular clinical use [7].

References

1. Deán-Ben, X.L., et al.: Advanced optoacoustic methods for multiscale imaging of in vivo dynamics. Chem. Soc. Rev. **46**, 2158–2198 (2017)
2. Mandal, S., Deán-Ben, X.L., Razansky, D.: Visual quality enhancement in optoacoustic tomography using active contour segmentation priors. IEEE Trans. Med. Imaging **35**(10), 2209–2217 (2016)
3. Mandal, S., Viswanath, P., Yeshaswini, N., Deán-Ben, X., Razansky, D.: Multiscale edge detection and parametric shape modeling for boundary delineation in optoacoustic images. In: 37th Annual International Conference of the IEEE Engineering in Medicine and Biology Society (EMBC), Milan, pp. 707–710 (2015)
4. Frangi, A.F., et al.: Multiscale vessel enhancement filtering. In: Wells, W.M., Colchester, A., Delp, S. (eds.) MICCAI 1998. LNCS, vol. 1496, pp. 130–137. Springer, Heidelberg (2006). https://doi.org/10.1007/BFb0056195
5. Ermolayev, V., Dean-Ben, X.L., Mandal, S., Ntziachristos, V., Razansky, D.: Simultaneous visualization of tumour oxygenation, neovascularization and contrast agent perfusion by real-time three-dimensional optoacoustic tomography. Eur. Radiol. **26**(6), 1843–1851 (2015). https://doi.org/10.1007/s00330-015-3980-0
6. Mandal, S., Greenblatt, A.B., An, J.: Imaging intelligence: AI is transforming medical imaging across the imaging spectrum. IEEE Pulse **9**(5), 16–24 (2018). https://doi.org/10.1109/MPUL.2018.2857226
7. Upputuri, P.K., Pramanik, M.: Recent advances toward preclinical and clinical translation of photoacoustic tomography: a review. J. Biomed. Opt. **22**(4), 041006 (2016)

Bootstrap Model Selection for Estimating the Sum of Exponentially Damped Sinusoids

Marcela Niemczyk(✉)

Wrocław University of Science and Technology, Wybrzeże Wyspiańskiego 27, 50-370 Wrocław, Poland
marcela.niemczyk@pwr.edu.pl

Abstract. Model estimation is an important issue in signal processing since it enables to characterize the signal and to obtain some parameters providing information about its shape. An example of a model widely used in various fields of science is the sum of exponentially damped sinusoids. In this work, a new method for parameters estimation of such a model is proposed. This method uses nonlinear least squares together with Fourier transform to estimate parameters of the sum of damped sinusoids. For model order selection, a bootstrap method is utilized. First, the presented method is verified on simulated signals. The efficacy of model order selection is assessed for signals with a different set value of signal-to-noise (SNR) ratio. It is shown that for the models with orders from 2 to 7, the order was estimated correctly in all trials for SNR greater than 20 dB. If a proper model order is selected, the set values of signal parameters are included in the confidence intervals for parameters values, determined by the nonlinear least squares method. Afterward, the described method is used for modeling the event-related potential in magnetoencephalography (MEG) signal. The method gives good fitting results with R^2 values greater than 0.9, showing its potential in MEG signals modeling and the assessment of brain activity.

Keywords: Bootstrap · Model selection · Sum of damped sinusoids · Magnetoencephalography

1 Introduction

The idea of signal modeling is to represent the signal by some model parameters. Models should be well-fitted to the signal, but simultaneously they should be also as simple as possible. An example of a model found in many fields of science is the sum of exponentially damped sinusoids. It is often used in spectroscopy [1,2], electroencephalography (EEG) [3,4], electric power systems [5], and also for audio signals modeling [6,7].

There are many different methods described in the literature for parameter estimation of the sum of damped sinusoids. Gillard and Kvasov have proposed a general nonlinear regression model [8], Kumaresan and Tufts were involving

N. Piaseczna et al. (Eds.): EMBS ICS 2020, AISC 1360, pp. 79–86, 2022.
https://doi.org/10.1007/978-3-030-88976-0_11

a linear prediction model with singular value decomposition (SVD) [9], whereas Parthasarathy and Tufts were using Newton's method to obtain maximum-likelihood estimators of the parameters of the sum of damped sinusoids [10]. For modeling EEG signal with the sum of damped sinusoids and estimate its parameters, Demiralp et al. were also considering Prony's method [3].

The sum of damped sinusoids can be also utilized as a model of magnetoencephalography signals [11]. Magnetoencephalography (MEG) is a functional neuroimaging technique in which a magnetic field, induced by electrical currents occurring in the brain, is recorded. It can be used for the investigation of event-related potentials (ERP), i.e., potentials occurring in a specific part of the brain following a specified stimulus. One of the approaches to explain the origin of these potentials is that ERPs are generated as a result of the reorganization of spontaneous brain activity [12]. As they are considered a superimposition of phase-resetted signals from populations of neurons in the brain, the extraction of the parameters of the signal components seems to be an appropriable method of their analysis [13].

2 Materials and Methods

2.1 Model Estimation

The model estimated in this work is described by the formula:

$$y(t) = \sum_{k=1}^{K} A_k e^{-\gamma_k t} \sin(\omega_k t + \phi_t) + \epsilon(t) \tag{1}$$

where each of K components is characterized by 4 parameters: A_k – amplitude, ω_k – frequency, ϕ_k – phase, γ_k – damping ratio. The number of components K is another parameter to be estimated. In addition, white noise $\epsilon(t)$ is included in the model.

All calculations and analyses were performed in MATLAB (MathWorks, Inc. Natick, MA, USA).

Nonlinear Least Squares Method. Due to the nonlinear behavior of considered signals, nonlinear least squares method was chosen for parameters estimation [14]. Since it was necessary to determine in advance the number of components for each analyzed signal, models of order from 1 to 10 were considered. Setting the initial values of parameters has a significant impact on the accuracy of estimation using nonlinear least squares. For this reason, the Fourier transform was proposed for preliminary estimation of the amplitude, frequency, and phase values for each component. Peaks in the amplitude spectrum were first sorted in descending order due to the amplitude. Then, the first K peaks were considered, where K indicates the assumed number of components. Amplitude spectrum of Fourier transform provided information about the amplitudes and frequencies of the components, while the values of phase were determined from the phase spectrum for the designated frequencies. Nonlinear least squares estimation, using Levenberg–Marquardt algorithms, was then performed with the calculated parameters set as initial values.

Bootstrap Model Selection. Having models of order from 1 to 10 fitted to the analyzed signal, an important issue was how to choose the best model. Considering only some goodness-of-fit measures could lead to the selection of the model with the highest order, which may be overfitted, i.e., fit not only the signal but also some noise. Therefore, based on [15], bootstrap method was proposed to achieve proper model order selection.

A scheme of that method is presented in Fig. 1. First, the parameters of the analyzed signal $y(t)$ need to be estimated. Based on them, a new signal $\hat{y}(t)$ is generated and the residuals are calculated as the difference between these two signals. These residuals may be considered as a noise, which is assumed to be independent and identically distributed random variables with unknown distribution with zero mean and variance of σ^2. Due to that, the bootstrap samples $r_1^*, r_2^*, \ldots, r_B^*$ are generated by resampling from the properly rescaled vector of residuals. Having B bootstrap residuals samples, they are added to the model signal $\hat{y}(t)$ to obtain the bootstrap signals $y_1^*(t), \ldots, y_B^*(t)$. The model is estimated for each of these signals and the sum of squared errors (SSE) is computed for the difference between these models and the original signal. For all tested model orders $k \in [1, 10]$, mean values of SSEs were set as $\Gamma(k)$ function values.

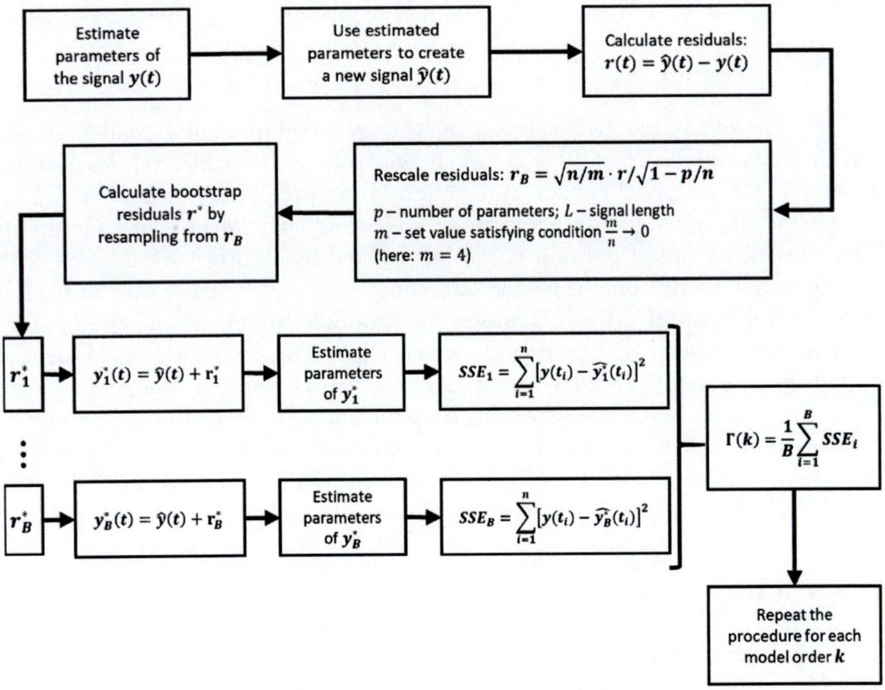

Fig. 1. A scheme of the bootstrap method for model selection

A linear penalty function was added to the Γ function to reduce the possibility to choose a model order that is too high. The minimum value of the sum of Γ

and penalty functions indicate the optimal (in the bootstrap sense) order of the model.

2.2 Simulated Signals

The proposed algorithm for the estimation of the model of exponentially damped sinusoids was first tested on simulated signals. Signals were generated for the chosen number of components and set values of amplitude, frequency, phase, and damping ratio for each of the components. For the simulated signal, white noise with different values of variance was added to obtain a set signal-to-noise ratio (SNR), defined as:

$$\mathrm{SNR} = 10\log_{10}\left(\frac{P_s}{P_n}\right)[dB] \tag{2}$$

where: P_s – the power of the signal, P_n – the power of noise.

To evaluate the efficacy of the proposed methods, signals of orders from 2 to 8 were generated with SNR values from 0 to 80 dB with a step of 10 dB. For each SNR value, the model estimation was repeated 10 times and the number of properly estimated models was calculated.

2.3 MEG Signal

The last part of this work considers using the proposed method of model estimation for MEG signals. Here, illustrative signals from one healthy adult subject are presented. The analyzed signals were acquired in Special Laboratory for Noninvasive Brain Imaging, Leibnitz Institute for Neurobiology, Magdeburg, Germany. They were containing the brain potentials evoked by auditory stimulation with the sinusoidal 1-kHz tone, repeated 224 times with a repetition rate of 0.5 Hz. After the rejection of artifacts, caused, for example, by eyeblinks, the number of trials was reduced to 190. Signals were acquired from 148 channels located around the head using a whole-head MEG system (4D-Neuroimaging, San Diego, USA). To reduce the noise, signals from each channel were averaged over all trials, as was described in [16]. The M100 potential, which presents the evoked potential occurring at about 100 ms after stimulation, was modeled. Signals from the channels with the highest amplitudes were selected for the analysis.

3 Results

3.1 Simulated Signals

Applying the proposed method of model estimation gave the model order and estimated values of model parameters together with their confidence intervals, calculated using nonlinear least squares method and the bootstrap. Performed analysis showed that if the model order was chosen correctly, the confidence intervals always contained the set values of parameters of the simulated signal.

However, the confidence intervals became wider with increasing noise (decreasing SNR values).

Figure 2 presents the fraction of correctly selected model orders in 10 trials for SNR values from 0 to 80 dB. It shows that 100% efficiency of model order selection was gained for signals with SNR values greater than: 30 dB for model order 8, 20 dB for model orders from 5 to 7, and 15 dB for model orders from 2 to 4.

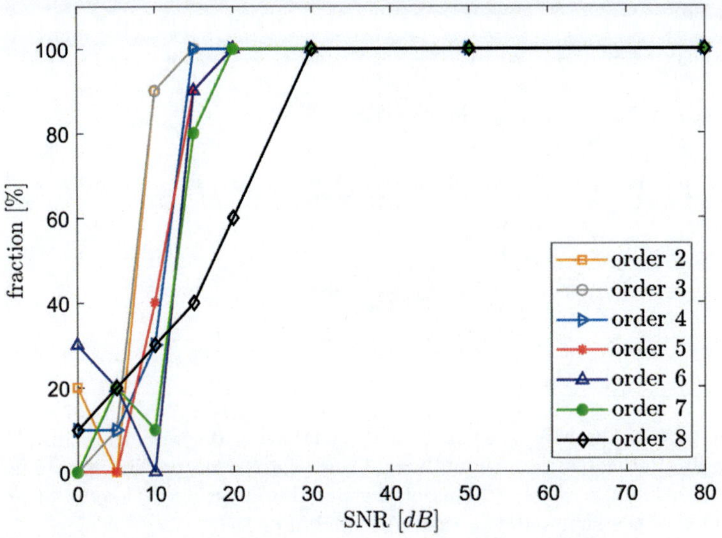

Fig. 2. Fractions of correctly calculated model orders in 10 trials performed for simulated signals with orders from 2 to 8 and SNR values from 0 to 80 dB.

3.2 MEG Signal

The proposed method of model selection was first applied for MEG signal from the channel with the highest amplitude (channel 110). It revealed that for this signal, with a length of 400 ms, the optimal model was of order 7. The fitting was evaluated using the coefficient of determination (R^2) and it gave R^2 value of 0.9328. Figure 3a shows that the signal contained not only the M100 peak but also the spontaneous brain activity (from 200 to 400 ms). To enhance the model fitting, the first 200 ms of the signal were considered (Fig. 3b). For such a signal, the estimated model was of order 3 and the M100 peak fitting was better, confirmed by the R^2 value of 0.9964.

Next, models for MEG signals from 10 other channels were also fitted. Signals with amplitudes greater than 250 fT were chosen for the analysis as they contained a pronounced M100 peak. The length of 200 ms was set for these signals. Using the proposed method of model estimation, models of orders 3 or 4 were selected to be optimal and $R^2 > 0.9$ was obtained for all analyzed signals.

4 Discussion

In this work, a new approach for modeling the sum of exponentially damped sinusoids was presented. Testing it on simulated signals revealed that this method effectively estimates the model when the level of noise is not high (SNR > 30 dB). It is worth noting that the estimation was performed for signals of orders up to 8, whereas in the literature simulations are often presented for a small number of components (see, e.g., [17,18]).

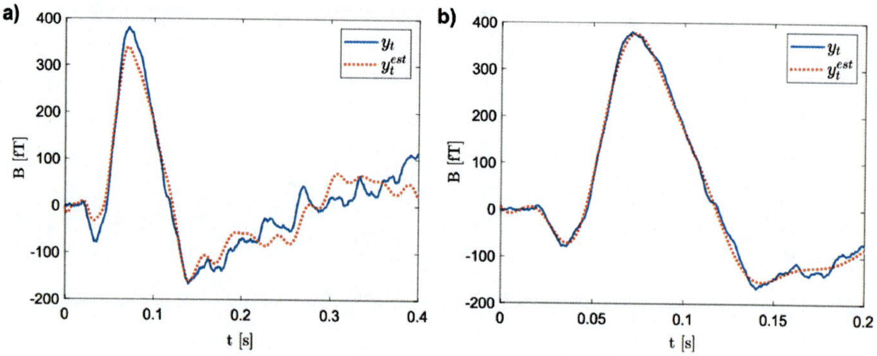

Fig. 3. A part of the MEG signal from the channel 110, presenting the M100 peak. The blue line indicates the original signal and the red dotted line presents a model selected as optimal. a) First 400 ms of the signal and estimated model of order 7; b) First 200 ms of the signal and estimated model of order 3.

The main limitation of this method is a considerable computation time. It is mainly caused by using the bootstrap method, which requires many repetitions of the model fitting. However, this bootstrap model selection is essential since the proper choice of the order is crucial for parameters estimation. Another limitation is that only a few illustrative MEG signals were considered, showing only the potential of the proposed method but not its suitability for this application in a general sense. Moreover, it is difficult to validate the correctness of the estimation as there are no certain methods for MEG signal estimation to compare with. For that reason, only the goodness-of-fit, assessed using R^2 value, was evaluated.

Testing the proposed method on ten MEG signals revealed that orders of the fitted models did not vary remarkably for signals coming from one subject but from different channels. Although the estimation method was applied only for a few MEG signals, it showed good fitting results and potential in the characterization of the signal components, worth to be explored in future research. Determining the parameters of the MEG signal may give valuable information about the brain activity and possible neurological disorders, increasing the diagnostic capabilities of this examination.

Acknowledgement. The author thanks D. Robert Iskander for his support and supervision at all stages of this work, and Cezary Sieluzycki for his help with MEG signals.

References

1. Duda, K., Magalas, L.B., Majewski, M., Zieliński, T.P.: DFT-based estimation of damped oscillation parameters in low-frequency mechanical spectroscopy. IEEE Trans Instrum Meas **60**, 3608–3618 (2011). https://doi.org/10.1109/TIM.2011.2113124
2. Umesh, S., Tufts, D.W.: Estimation of parameters of exponentially damped sinusoids using fast maximum likelihood estimation with application to NMR spectroscopy data. IEEE Trans. Signal Process. **44**, 2245–2259 (1996). https://doi.org/10.1109/78.536681
3. Demiralp, T., Ademoglu, A., Istefanopulos, Y., Gülçür, H.Ö.: Analysis of event-related potentials (ERP) by damped sinusoids. Biol. Cybern. **78**, 487–493 (1998). https://doi.org/10.1007/s004220050452
4. Franaszczuk, P.J., Blinowska, K.J.: Linear model of brain electrical activity-EEG as a superposition of damped oscillatory modes. Biol. Cybern. **53**, 19–25 (1985). https://doi.org/10.1007/BF00355687
5. Lovisolo, L., da Silva, E.A.B., Rodrigues, M.A.M., Diniz, P.S.R.: Efficient coherent adaptive representations of monitored electric signals in power systems using damped sinusoids. IEEE Trans. Signal Process. **53**, 3831–3846 (2005). https://doi.org/10.1109/TSP.2005.855400
6. Hermus, K., Verhelst, W., Lemmerling, P., et al.: Perceptual audio modeling with exponentially damped sinusoids. Signal Process. **85**, 163–176 (2005). https://doi.org/10.1016/j.sigpro.2004.09.010
7. Nieuwenhuijse, J., Heusens, R., Deprettere, E.F.: Robust exponential modeling of audio signals. In: ICASSP, IEEE International Conference on Acoustics, Speech and Signal Processing - Proceedings, pp. 3581–3584. Institute of Electrical and Electronics Engineers Inc. (1998)
8. Gillard, J.W., Kvasov, D.E.: Lipschitz optimization methods for fitting a sum of damped sinusoids to a series of observations. Stat Interface **10**, 59–70 (2017). https://doi.org/10.4310/SII.2017.v10.n1.a6
9. Kumaresan, R., Tufts, D.W.: Estimating the parameters of exponentially damped sinusoids and pole-zero modeling in noise. IEEE Trans. Acoust. **30**, 833–840 (1982). https://doi.org/10.1109/TASSP.1982.1163974
10. Parthasarathy, S., Tufts, D.W.: Maximum-likelihood estimation of parameters of exponentially damped sinusoids. Proc. IEEE **73**, 1528–1530 (1985). https://doi.org/10.1109/PROC.1985.13328
11. Gopalakrishnan, R., Machado, A.G., Burgess, R.C., Mosher, J.C.: The use of contact heat evoked potential stimulator (CHEPS) in magnetoencephalography for pain research. J. Neurosci. Methods **220**, 55–63 (2013). https://doi.org/10.1016/j.jneumeth.2013.08.015
12. Savers, B., Beagley, H.A., Henshall, W.R.: The mechanism of auditory evoked EEG responses. Nature **247**, 481–483 (1974). https://doi.org/10.1038/247481a0
13. Basar, E.: Toward a physical approach to integrative physiology. I. Brain dynamics and physical causality. Am. J. Physiol. Regul. Integr. Comp. Physiol. **245**, R513–R533 (1983). https://doi.org/10.1152/ajpregu.1983.245.4.r510

14. Quinn, B.G.: On fitting exponentially damped sinusoids. In: IEEE Workshop on Statistical Signal Processing Proceedings, pp. 201–204 (2014)
15. Zoubir, A.M., Iskander, D.R.: Bootstrap Techniques for Signal Processing. Cambridge University Press, Cambridge (2004)
16. Sieluzycki, C., König, R., Matysiak, A., et al.: Single-trial evoked brain responses modeled by multivariate matching pursuit. IEEE Trans. Biomed. Eng. **56**, 74–82 (2009). https://doi.org/10.1109/TBME.2008.2002151
17. Papadopoulos, C.K., Nikias, C.L.: Parameter estimation of exponentially damped sinusoids using higher order statistics. IEEE Trans. Acoust. **38**, 1424–1436 (1990). https://doi.org/10.1109/29.57577
18. Chan, F.K.W., So, H.C., Sun, W.: Subspace approach for two-dimensional parameter estimation of multiple damped sinusoids. Signal Process. **92**, 2172–2179 (2012). https://doi.org/10.1016/j.sigpro.2012.02.003

Tracking the Local Backscatter Changes in Cornea Scheimpflug Images During Tonometry Measurement with OCULUS Corvis ST

Maria Miażdżyk(✉)

Wrocław University of Science and Technology, Wybrzeże Wyspiańskiego 27, 50-370 Wrocław, Poland
maria.miazdzyk@pwr.edu.pl

Abstract. The purpose of this study was to track the local backscatter changes in cornea Scheimpflug images observed during tonometry measurements with OCULUS Corvis ST. 10 healthy-eyed adult measurement results were used and, from every measurement, 140 cornea images were obtained. Initially, corneal edge detection was performed. Subsequently, the cornea was segmented into small, linear sections, perpendicular to the corneal curvature. That allowed for pixel intensity averaging of each section. As a result, colormaps with mean pixel intensity for every section and every frame were received. Finally, in 8 out of 10 colormaps the strongest backscatter local changes were visible.

Keywords: Cornea · Tonometry · Scheimpflug camera · Local backscatter changes · Image processing

1 Introduction

Corvis ST (Oculus Optikgerate, Inc., Wetzlar, Germany) is an "air puff" noncontact tonometer for intraocular pressure (IOP) measurements. Additionally, it provides the means for calculating parameters related to corneal biomechanics. Corvis ST is equipped with a high-speed Scheimpflug camera that collects 4330 frames per second during ca. 30 ms of examination. Applied gaussian-like air impulse provokes the corneal deformation response, which is recorded (Fig. 1). As a result, Corvis ST returns almost 40 anatomical and biomechanical parameters such as, to mention just a few, intraocular pressure (IOP), central corneal thickness (CCT), deformation amplitude (DA) and Corneal Biomechanical Index (CBI). Despite useful macro parameters calculated purely by Corvis ST software for edge detection, there are some studies that perform analysis of the stromal backscatter distribution recorded in Scheimpflug images to inquire corneal microstructure characteristics and improve diagnostics of corneal disorders such as keratoconus or glaucoma [1–3]. It was also demonstrated that speckle distribution in corneal optical coherence tomography (OCT) is related to corneal tissue properties at micro scale [4–6]. This novel course of research encourages to explore new opportunities for corneal image processing and image statistical analysis.

N. Piaseczna et al. (Eds.): EMBS ICS 2020, AISC 1360, pp. 87–93, 2022.
https://doi.org/10.1007/978-3-030-88976-0_12

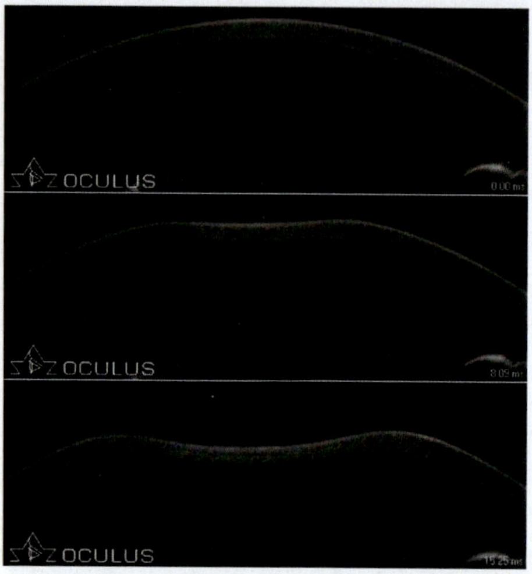

Fig. 1. An example of three Scheimpflug images from a 30 ms Corvis ST measurement. From top to bottom: cornea image at time 0.0 ms, 8.09 ms, and at 15.25 ms.

2 Purpose

During Corvis ST measurement, some changes in the corneal backscatter, corresponding to changes in local pixel intensity, were observed (Fig. 2). Between the 40–60th frame of measurement, in the off-central parts of the cornea, some high intensity lines can be perceived. These lines are approximately perpendicular to the corneal curvature and migrate to the peripheral sides due to measurement progress. The aforementioned observation encouraged the author to carry out an image analysis that would effectively exhibit the process of local pixel intensity changes.

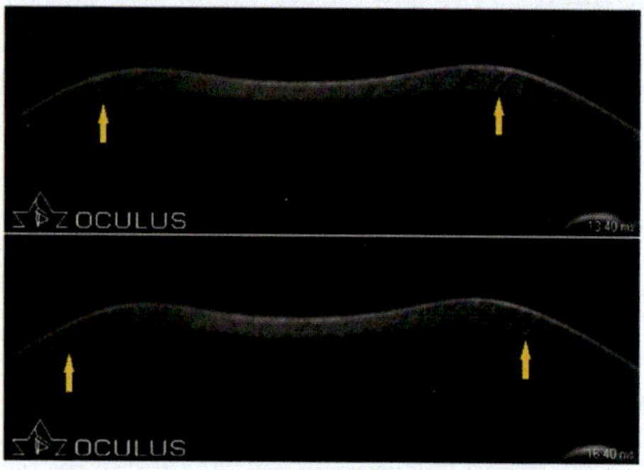

Fig. 2. Bright lines observed in cornea Scheimpflug images during Corvis ST measurement: cornea at 13.40 ms (top) and at 16.40 ms (bottom). Yellow arrows indicate the localization of the observed phenomenon.

3 Methods

3.1 Data

10 Corvis ST examination results acquired with the consent of Consejo et al. [3] were included. More detailed information about Corvis ST data acquisition is explained in [3]. Patients were healthy-eyed adults, aged between 18–29 years old.

3.2 Image Analysis

Initially, every single 30 ms measurement (eye was chosen randomly) was exported from Corvis ST software and, for every patient, a 140-frame set of cornea Scheimpflug images was received. Images were of size 200×576 pixels and had an approximate resolution of 15 μm/pixel horizontally and 24 μm/pixel vertically. The whole subsequent picture analysis was performed in Matlab (version R2020b, MathWorks, Natick, MA, USA), the summary of consecutive steps is shown in Fig. 3. The first stage of image processing was corneal edge detection, for which the algorithm proposed in [3] was employed. The main operations for this algorithm were median filter and Canny edge detection. The concept of local pixel intensity tracking comprised of corneal segmentation into small linear sections, perpendicular to the corneal curvature. The following analysis required fitting a function to the detected edges. The 8th order polynomial proved to be the best fit due to the fact that the cornea in the concave state has 3 local extremes. Goodness-of-fit (GOF) was evaluated visually. None of the images (with correct edge detection) showed overfitting. To exclude the epithelium, which is brighter and carries different information than the stroma, 8-pixel margin was set (Fig. 4).

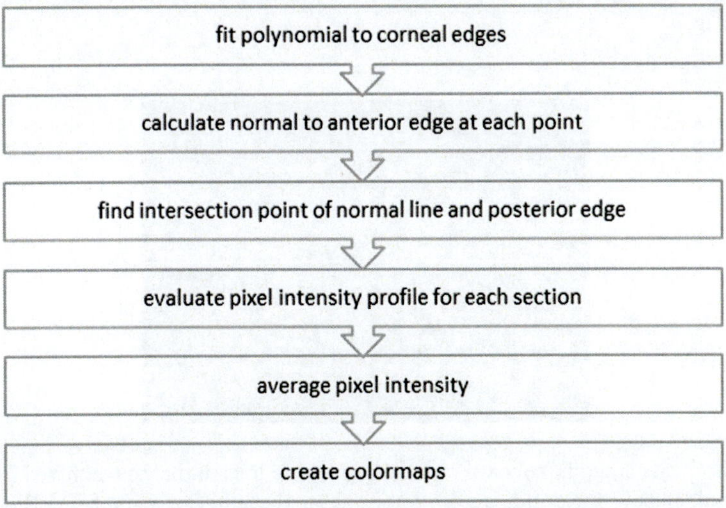

Fig. 3. Summary of performed image analysis.

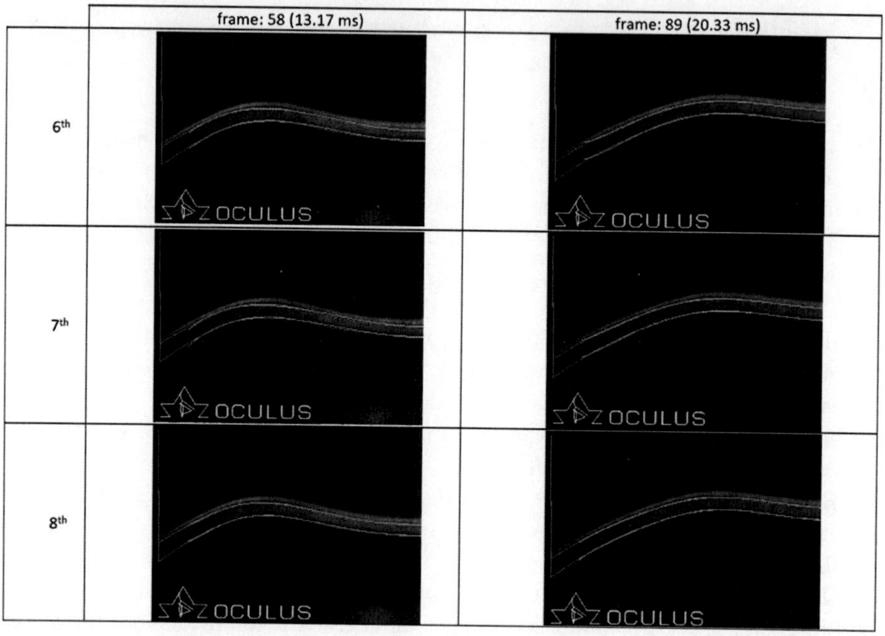

Fig. 4. Polynomial fitting to corneal edges. Bright line indicates the fitted function, red line – detected edges. Left column of the table includes polynomial order. For the anterior edge 8-pixel epithelium margin is excluded. Finally, the 8th order polynomial was chosen.

Subsequently, for each point of the anterior edge, a normal line was calculated, then the intersection point for the posterior edge and the normal was found (Fig. 5).

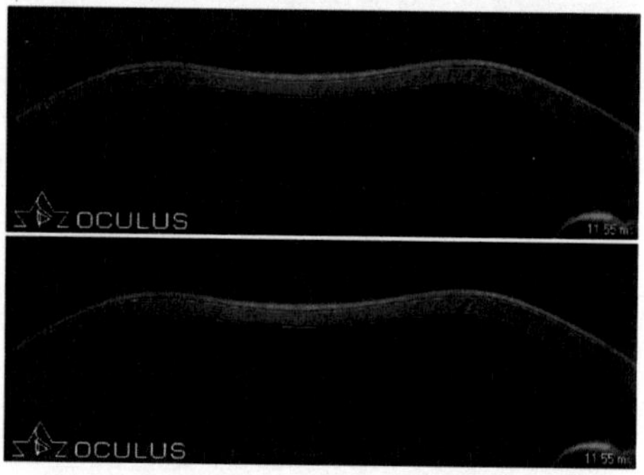

Fig. 5. Corneal image in concave state. Bright blue lines indicate the fitted 8th order polynomial, purple lines indicate the normal to the anterior curvature. Blue circles indicate the beginning and the end of chosen section.

Mean pixel intensity for each section was computed with the use of Matlab improfile function. The improfile function, independently from the input section length, returns a vector with a fixed size (set as an input argument) including interpolated (nearest neighbours method) pixel intensity values. The length of the vector was fixed for 25 pixels, and every single result was averaged. That allowed for the construction of colormaps with mean pixel intensity at each section in each frame of examination (Fig. 6).

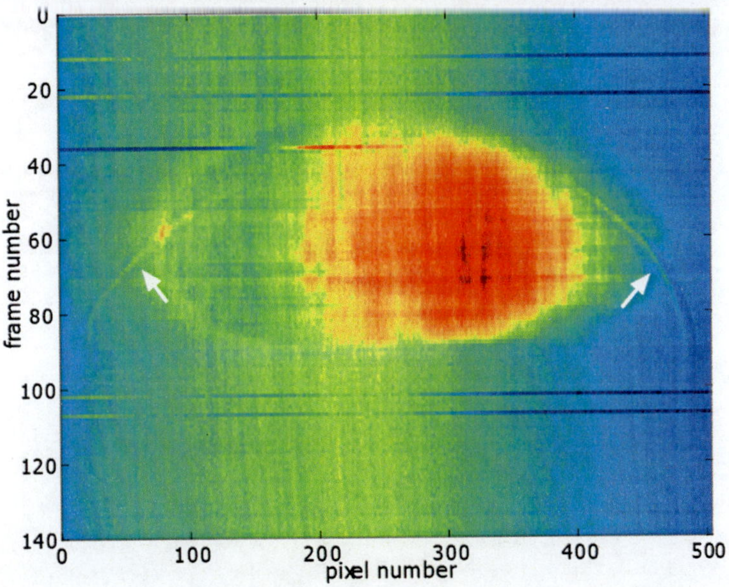

Fig. 6. Colormap generated for one patient. Image indicates mean pixel intensity for every single section of cornea (x), for every frame (y). White arrow indicates visible migrating peak.

Colormaps were processed to highlight the local intensity changes and exclude global lightening of the cornea caused by its concavity. To normalize the graphs, it was necessary to subtract a constant equal to the nonzero minimum of the mean pixel intensity matrix, and then divide it by the maximum value. Another operation was the moving average (window size: 25) subtraction (Fig. 7).

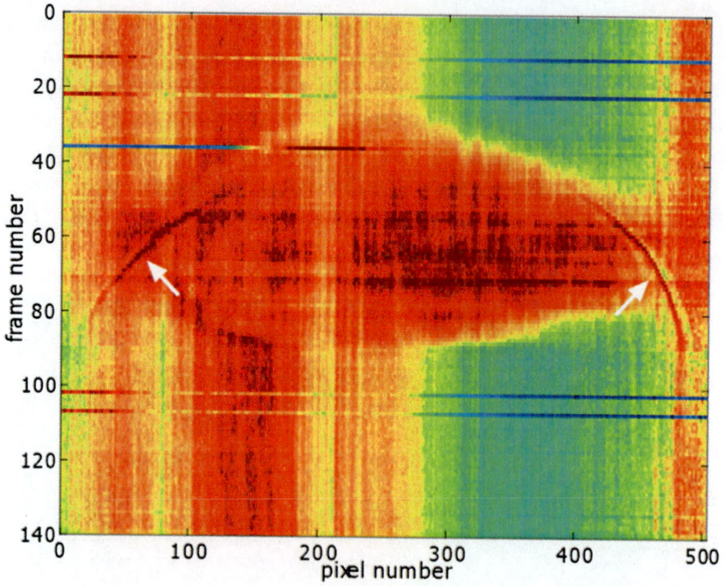

(a)

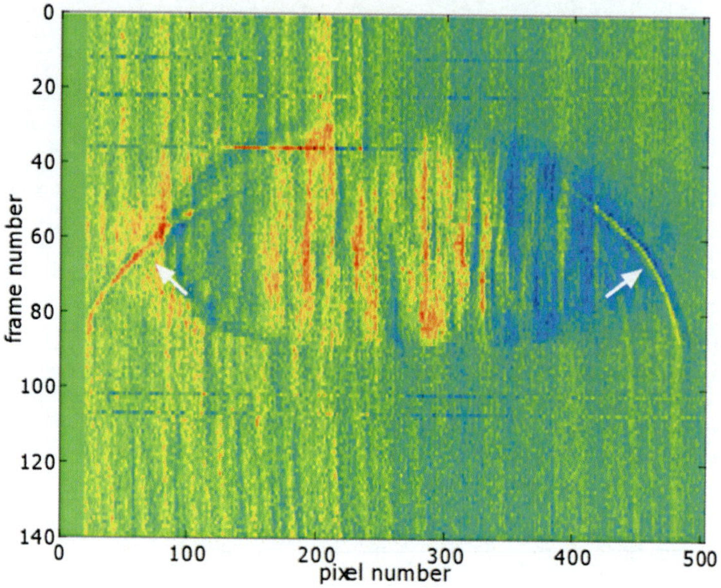

(b)

Fig. 7. Processed colormaps generated for one patient – a) normalized colormap, b) colormap with subtracted moving average. Images indicate mean pixel intensity for every single section of cornea (x), for every frame (y).

4 Summary

The performed analysis allowed for tracking the migrating peak in 8 out of 10 results. In the remaining 2 cases, although low-contrast migrating peaks were noticeable in the image data, they were not trackable in colormaps. In some colormaps also lower intensity backscatter changes were visible (2 out of 10), however, to observe them more precisely, an improved analysis would be necessary. Another issue could be raised regarding the origin of migrating peaks and the process of propagation. Presumably, the peaks represent a kind of longitudinal mechanical wave induced by air impulse and corneal deformation. Hereby, further study is a proper step to inquire this point and extend the knowledge about corneal biomechanics.

References

1. Iskander, D.R., Consejo, A., Solarski, J., Karnowski, K., et al.: Corneal properties of Glaucoma based on Scheimpflug light intensity distribution. Invest. Ophthalmol. Vis. Sci. **61**(7), 4716 (2020)
2. Consejo, A., Solarski, J., Karnowski, K., Rozema, J.J., et al.: Keratoconus detection based on a single Scheimpflug image. Trans. Vis. Sci. Tech. **9**(7), 36 (2020)
3. Consejo, A., Gławdecka, K., Karnowski, K., Solarski, J., et al.: Corneal properties of keratoconus based on Scheimpflug light intensity distribution. Invest. Ophthalmol. Vis. Sci. **60**(8), 3197–3203 (2019)
4. Iskander, D.R., Kostyszak, M., Jesus, D., Majewska, M., et al.: Assessing corneal speckle in optical coherence tomography: a new look at glaucomatous eyes. Optom. Vis. Sci. **97**(2), 62–67 (2020)
5. Danielewska, M., Antończyk, A., Rogala, M., Jesus, D., et al.: Corneal OCT speckle differences in crosslinked and untreated rabbit eyes in response to elevated intraocular pressure. Invest. Ophthalmol. Vis. Sci. **61**(7), 4713 (2020)
6. Jesus, D., Iskander, D.R.: Assessment of corneal properties based on statistical modeling of OCT speckle. Biomed Opt Express. **8**, 162–176 (2017)

A Preliminary Approach to Plaque Detection in MRI Brain Images

Karolina Milewska[1], Rafał Obuchowicz[2], and Adam Piórkowski[1](✉)

[1] Department of Biocybernetics and Biomedical Engineering, AGH University of Science and Technology, Mickiewicza 30 Avenue, 30–059 Krakow, Poland
pioro@agh.edu.pl

[2] Department of Diagnostic Imaging, Jagiellonian University Medical College, Kopernika 19, 31–501 Krakow, Poland

Abstract. Demyelinating plaques are areas of perineural demyelination, i.e., areas where myelin has disappeared due to regional ischemia or autoimmune diseases; they are visible as white matter hyperintensities in MR imaging. Regional blood flow reduction provokes a state in which the metabolic needs of the neuron are not met. The aforementioned metabolic imbalance of the neuron is the most frequent causative factor of demyelination. Local thrombosis, small vessel disease, or vessel compression are possible causative factors that provoke regional ischemia. The autoimmune background is also a possible cause as it usually results in numerous foci in brain white matter and the spinal cord.

This article presents the experimental results of various algorithms applied for the segmentation of plaques. This issue is briefly discussed from a medical point of view, after which data obtained from magnetic resonance imaging, in particular from the Turbo Inversion Recovery Magnitude (TIRM) protocol, is shown. Then, experimental test results for convolutional filtering and a group of local binarization algorithms are presented. Algorithm sequences are also proposed that achieve an important increase in accuracy. The results are evaluated and the parameter spaces are defined for the best algorithms, including Sauvola, Local Normalization and SDA.

Keywords: Plaques · Cerebrum · Segmentation · Sauvola · Local normalization

1 Introduction

On the cellular level, lesions in brain white matter are actually myelin loss around axons. A plaque of demyelination is formed where myelin loss is present not only on the level of a single neuron but is also widespread in a larger group of neurons. Such lesions can be detected in MRI due to local changes in water content. In most cases, this is caused by a regional reduction of the blood flow when the metabolic needs of the neuron are not met. This state causes loss of myelin

N. Piaseczna et al. (Eds.): EMBS ICS 2020, AISC 1360, pp. 94–105, 2022.
https://doi.org/10.1007/978-3-030-88976-0_13

in the white matter or spinal cord, which is called nonspecific vascular-derived demyelination plaque. The most important disease entities are microangiopathy, polyangiopathy, and random infarcts. Small vessel disease is a known causative entity of numerous subcortical plaques that are possibly present in young age. On the other hand, there are demyelination autoimmune diseases which cause widespread myelin loss across the brain matter and may induce serious clinical disabilities and impairment of brain function. The most frequent and serious autoimmune disease is multiple sclerosis. If it occurs, demyelination foci can embrace a substantial area of the brain and spinal cord.

Regarding visual analysis of multiple sclerosis plaques, they can be much more hyperintense on MRI images in comparison to the plaques caused by vascular disease, especially in an acute state of sclerosis multiplex, which may induce edema of neural tissue. In both cases, segmenting and detecting these changes is not trivial because they have irregular shape and size and their intensity varies. This detection difficulty is evident in the case of vascular plaques, which are challenging to distinguish from the white matter background even for experienced radiologists. Importantly, in most cases demyelination is detected on the basis of a signal change in T2-weighted sequences (with dominant transverse - a "spin-spin" relaxation), i.e. FLAIR in an imaging protocol. Importantly, they are hypertensive in T2-weighted sequences, i.e., the FLAIR MRI imaging protocol.

Similar studies were recently presented in [1]. In this article, automatic and semi-automatic lesion-detection algorithms were tested that were based on existing literature, e.g., region growing and neural network solutions. According to these authors' conclusions, the most accurate algorithms in this case are Convolution Neural Networks and Deep Learning methods.

In [2], Ilkay Oksuz also proposed the use of Convolution Neural Networks based on Densetnet-201. Theoretically, Densetnet-201 gave results with the precision of c.a. 0.97, but in contrast to our work, artefacts in MRI images were generated synthetically. On the basis of the presented research, further analysis of plaque-detection techniques is needed. Practical semi- or fully automatic application of plaque-detection algorithms will support radiologists [3].

2 Materials and Methods

2.1 The Dataset

The dataset contains 3 examples of 12-bit DICOM images of brain MRI in TIRM mode (Fig. 1). For the analysis, the images were reduced by scaling to 8-bit depth. Images were acquired using three types of MRI scanners: Magnetom Essenza, Avanto Fit and Skyra (3T). The resolution of the images is also different: in the presented dataset, the values are, respectively 0.71875×0.71875, 0.375×0.375 and 0.859375×0.859375 (Table 1). The ROI, which depicts white matter, was segmented by a semi-automatic method, and the plaques were marked on the pictures manually.

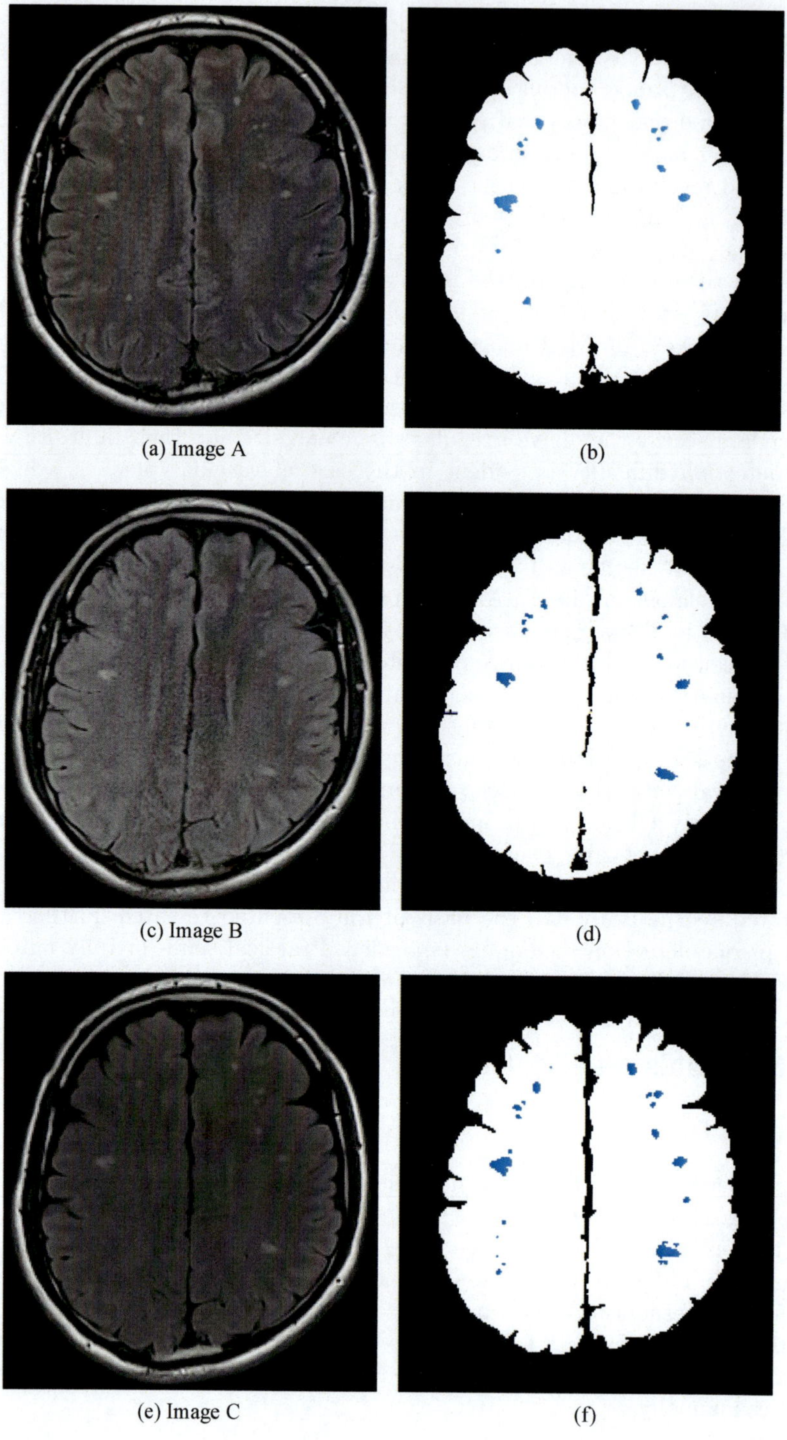

Fig. 1. Images presented in the article and theirs ROI.

Table 1. Image properities.

ID	Scanner model	Pixel spacing	Original matrix (px)
A	Avanto	0.375 × 0.375	540 × 640
B	Magnetom Essenza	0.71875 × 0.71875	252 × 320
C	Skyra (3T)	0.859375 × 0.859375	256 × 256

2.2 Binarization

A few algorithms were tested in the first part of the research to determine if they could be used for lesion detection: global thresholding and nuclei-segmentation algorithms seemed to be promising, but finally it turned out that they do not produce any acceptable results. Neither the Nuclei Counter from Matlab File Exchange nor the use of neural networks [4,5] delivered satisfactory results.

Hough Transform (elliptic and circle) and Radial Symmetry Transform (RST) also did not detect plaques satisfactorily, mainly because both focused on regular round structures, but plaques have irregular shapes and they are often smaller than cells in microscopic images. Hough Transform was checked using the OpenCV Python library, and RST was checked with the ImageJ plugin [6,7].

Convolution filtering was also tested. In the case of plaque detection, it indicated the location of plaques, but it did not do so precisely. Examples of an image and a mask are shown in Fig. 2.

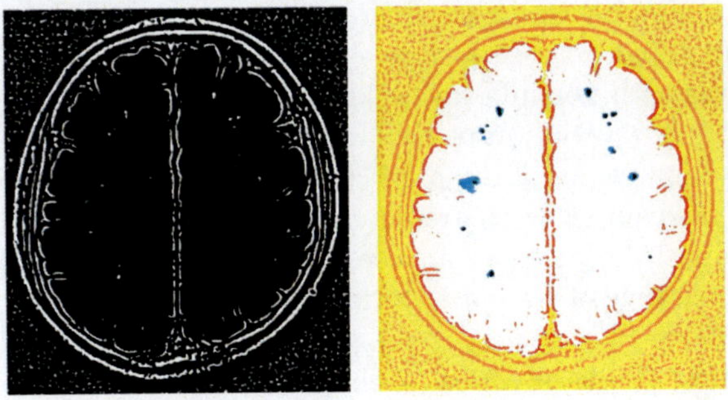

-3	-3	-2	-2	-2	-2	-2	-3	-3
-3	-2	-1	-1	-1	-1	-1	-2	-3
-2	-1	0	0	0	0	0	-1	-2
-2	-1	0	6	6	6	0	-1	-2
-2	-1	0	6	40	6	0	-1	-2
-2	-1	0	6	6	6	0	-1	-2
-2	-1	0	0	0	0	0	-1	-2
-3	-2	-1	-1	-1	-1	-1	-2	-3
-3	-3	-2	-2	-2	-2	-2	-3	-3

Fig. 2. Image A - an example result of convolutional filter.

The next approach was to test a group of well-known segmentation algorithms that are implemented in the ImageJ and Matlab environments. Global and local thresholding was taken into account. Both automatic and manual global thresholding did not produce the expected results because they did not show all plaques; moreover, the output images contained various random objects and other structures.

2.3 Local Thresholding Algorithms

Local thresholding is based on binarization in the local environment for each pixel independently. Most often, a circle-shaped neighborhood of a pixel is chosen. During this research, the following thresholding methods were tested: Contrast, Bernsen, Mean, Median, Midgrey, Otsu, Niblack, Sauvola, Phansalkar, Local Normalization and the Statistical Dominance Algorithm.

The final tests showed that the combination of LN and SDA achieves the best precision for plaque segmentation.

Contrast Thresholding sets a positive pixel value when the current value is closer to the local maximum; otherwise, it sets a negative value. Kernel radius is the one parameter that should be set by the user [8]. This method did not provide satisfactory results in the context of plaque detection.

Bernsen's method uses the circular-shaped context of a pixel. Two user parameters need to be set for this algorithm: radius and contrast threshold [9,10].

Mean Local Threshold also provides two parameters (radius and C-value). C is a constant and its default value is 0. The mean of the local greyscale distribution is selected as the threshold in this case.

Median – instead of the mean threshold, this takes a median of the local greyscale distribution. The additional parameter is also a C-value.

MidGray Thresholding selects the mid-grey of the same element as the previous two methods.

Otsu takes the threshold minimizing weighted sum of variances of the two classes. In this case, instead of global Otsu, pixels are verified in regions. Kernel radius is the only user-provided parameter [11].

Niblack Threshold is a method which uses three parameters: r - radius, k-value (with 0.2 as a default), and offset, which is a C-value in this case (0 is default). It is useful for images with nonuniform backgrounds [12].

Sauvola's Method – this is a variation of Niblack thresholding that gives very interesting results, with high values of the precision coefficient. Apart from the kernel radius (r), Sauvola requires two parameters: k-value (which amplifies the contribution of standard deviation in an adaptive manner with 0.5 as default), and r-value (dynamic range of standard deviation, with 128 as default) [13].

Phansalkar Thresholding [14] is intended for low-contrast images. It is a modification of the Sauvola method. This technique was not tested for plaque segmentation because it uses four parameters, therefore adjusting them is highly complex. The r-value is different than the one from Sauvola; here it is the normalized intensity of the image.

Statistical Dominance Algorithm (SDA) – interesting algorithm for lesion detection [15], which is designed for small object detection [16,17]. It promotes small objects in disc-shaped areas (radius $SDAr$) that are contrasted against the background by at least a given threshold ($SDAt$).

Local Normalization (NA) – additionally, the brightness of small objects can be enhanced using Local Normalization [18]. To achieve satisfactory results, it is necessary to properly define two parameters: sigma to estimate the local mean ($sigma1$), and sigma to estimate the local variance ($sigma2$).

3 Results

The test scripts were processed in ImageJ (v. 1.53 g) [19,20]. The best set of parameters was sought for each algorithm using two PCs (Intel i9-7900X and AMD 3800X equipped), in a similar way as is presented in [21]. The preliminary tests excluded algorithms that gave no acceptable results. Further investigation revealed which three of the presented algorithms were best in the context of precise segmentation.

3.1 SDA

Preliminary tests with available SDA neighborhoods were first performed (disc, snowflake and their normalized versions); this revealed that the best values are achieved for the normalized disc mode (round neighborhood), so the next analysis was done only for that one. The highest Dice coefficient values for SDA were close to 0.55 (Table 2). Figure 3 shows the relation between the $SDAr$ and the $SDAt$ parameters for the best Dice values.

Table 2. Results for tested algorithms for A, B and C images, where Dice coefficient higher than 0.1.

Image	Algorithm	Settings	Best dice
A	Contrast	r = 63	0.1505
	Midgray	r = 66, c = –25	0.2154
	Mean	r = 48, c = –25	0.2583
	Median	r = 16, c = –21	0.3194
	SDA	sdar = 25, sdat = 14, binth = 198	0.4865
	Sauvola	r = 51, kv = 015, rv = 2.45	0.6158
	LN + SDA	sigma1 = 24, sigma2 = 22, sdar = 23, sdat = 30	0.6468
B	SDA	sdar = 14, sdat = 17, binth = 217	0.4532
	Sauvola	r =26, kv = 0.25, rv = 3.95	0.5185
	LN + SDA	sigma1 = 9, sigma2 = 11, sdar = 12, sdat = 40	0.6032
C	SDA	sdar = 18, sdat = 5, binth = 234	0.5566
	Sauvola	r = 15, kv = –0.05, rv = –1.15	0.6097
	LN + SDA	sigma1 = 10, sigma2 = 8, sdar=11, sdat = 25	**0.699**

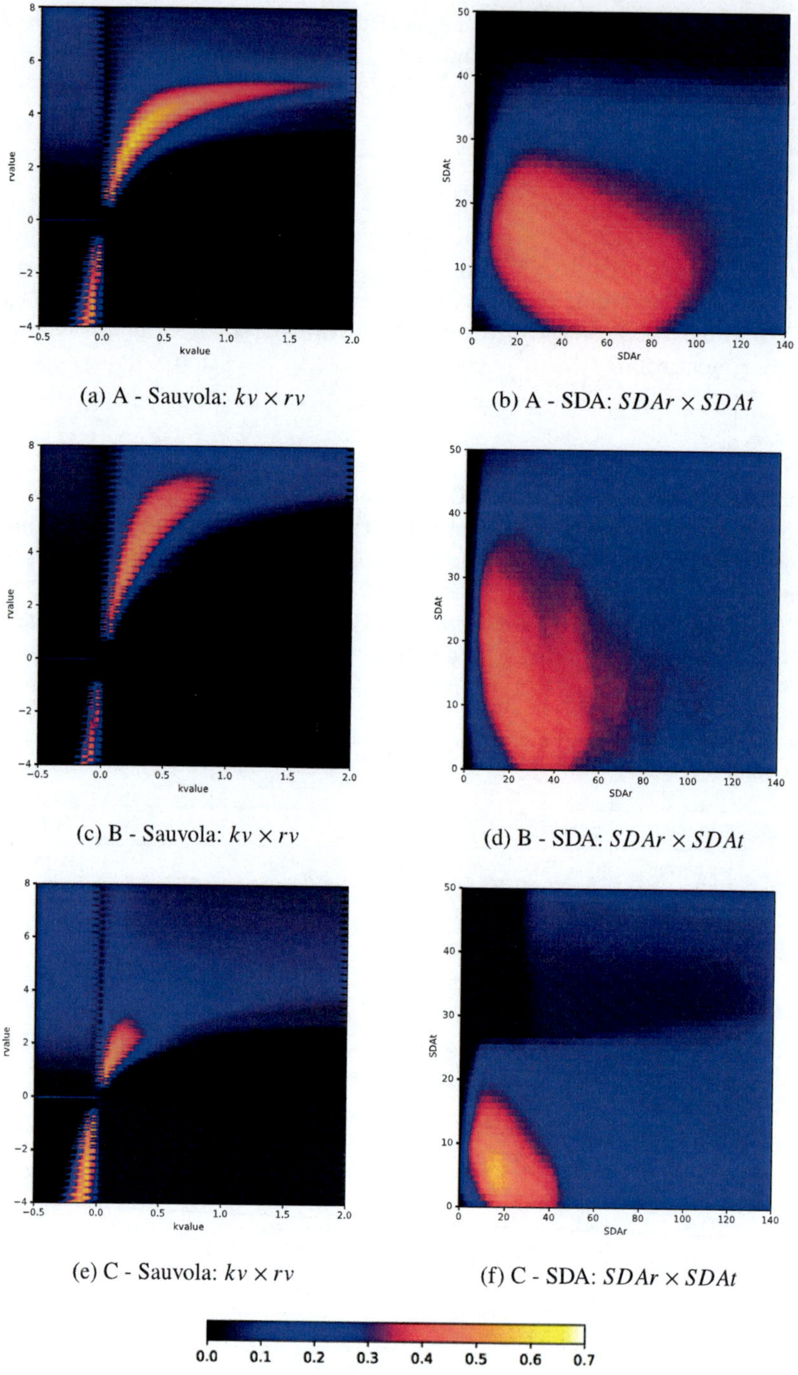

(a) A - Sauvola: $kv \times rv$

(b) A - SDA: $SDAr \times SDAt$

(c) B - Sauvola: $kv \times rv$

(d) B - SDA: $SDAr \times SDAt$

(e) C - Sauvola: $kv \times rv$

(f) C - SDA: $SDAr \times SDAt$

(g) color scale for Dice values

Fig. 3. Parameters space of Sauvola and SDA algorithms for images A, B, and C.

3.2 Sauvola Local Thresholding

For this kind of thresholding, surprising results were obtained because the precision of plaque detection was close to 0.6 (Table 2). This was higher than the SDA results. The parameter space was covered with a precision step of 0.05 for k-value and r-value, and with a step of 1 for radius. Figure 3 shows the highest Dice coefficient results for Sauvola, especially the relation between the r-value and the k-value. Figure 4 shows the dependencies between the radius and the Dice coefficient. After careful analysis of each image, it was found that there are no common optimal parameter values for the segmentation of all images, despite the fact that this group of algorithms is called "auto local threshold". Moreover, the highest Dice coefficient is reached when using r-value and k-value parameters that are completely different from the original default, especially when it comes to r-value ($rv = 128$), and even for negative values. This leads to the conclusion that despite the fact that this algorithm detects plaques with relatively high accuracy, it is not an algorithm that could lead to the development of a fully automatic method.

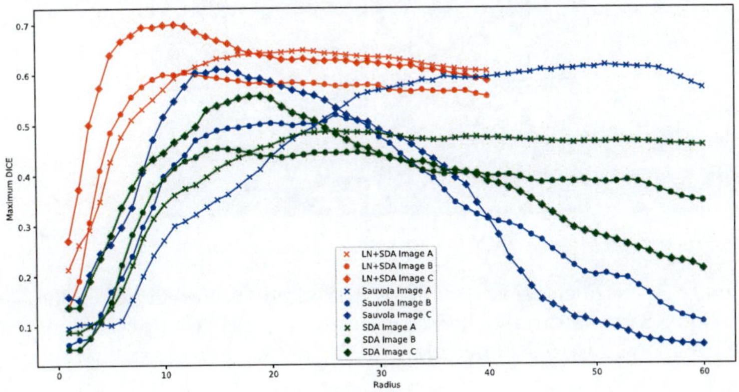

Fig. 4. Maximum dice coefficients depending on radius.

3.3 LN with SDA

As Local Normalization enhances the brightness of plaques, SDA should detect the lesions better (Fig. 5). A script task verified all parameters for a combination of these two algorithms: $sigma1$ and $sigma2$ for LN; $SDAr$ and $SDAt$ for SDA and final thresholding. Figure 6 shows the distribution of parameters separately for the LN and SDA algorithms to visualize the parameter space and find the best Dice values.

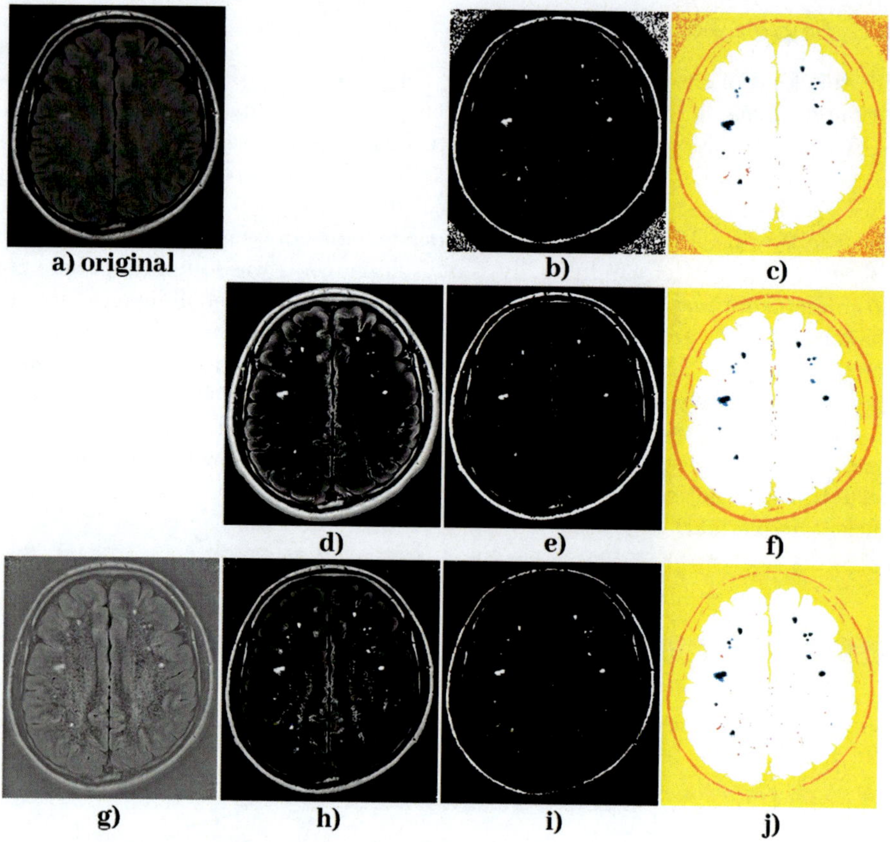

Fig. 5. Image A - segmentation results for maximum Dice coefficient values - original image (a), after Sauvola thresholding (b,c), after SDA (d) and thresholding (e,f), after LN (g), SDA (h) and thresholding (i,j).

3.4 Relation Between Radius and Pixel Spacing

The results were as expected: there is a direct relation between the best-solution radius and pixel spacing. Figure 7 shows the relations for Sauvola, SDA and LN+SDA. The higher the pixel spacing, the lower the radius values.

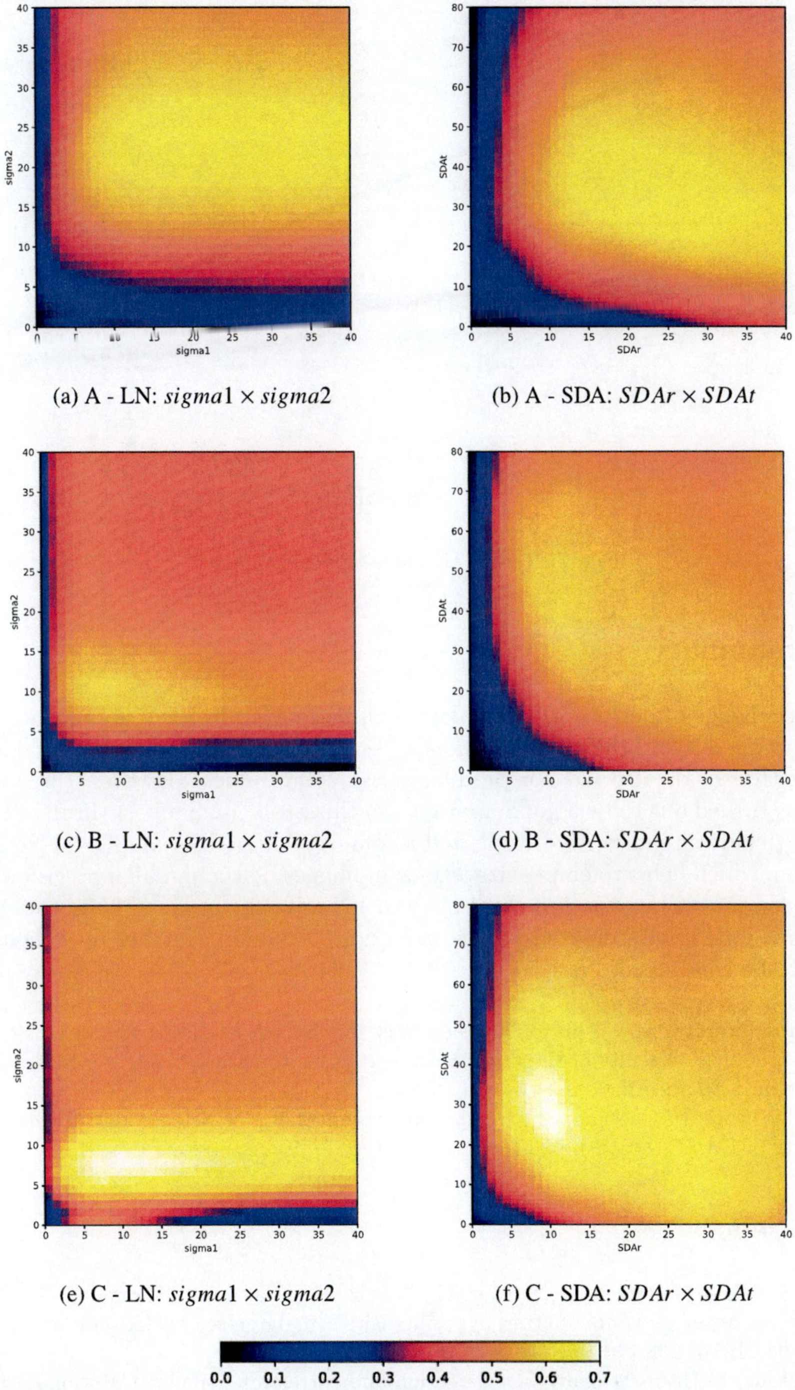

(a) A - LN: *sigma*1 × *sigma*2

(b) A - SDA: *SDAr* × *SDAt*

(c) B - LN: *sigma*1 × *sigma*2

(d) B - SDA: *SDAr* × *SDAt*

(e) C - LN: *sigma*1 × *sigma*2

(f) C - SDA: *SDAr* × *SDAt*

(g) color scale for Dice values

Fig. 6. Parameters space of LN and SDA combination for images A, B, and C.

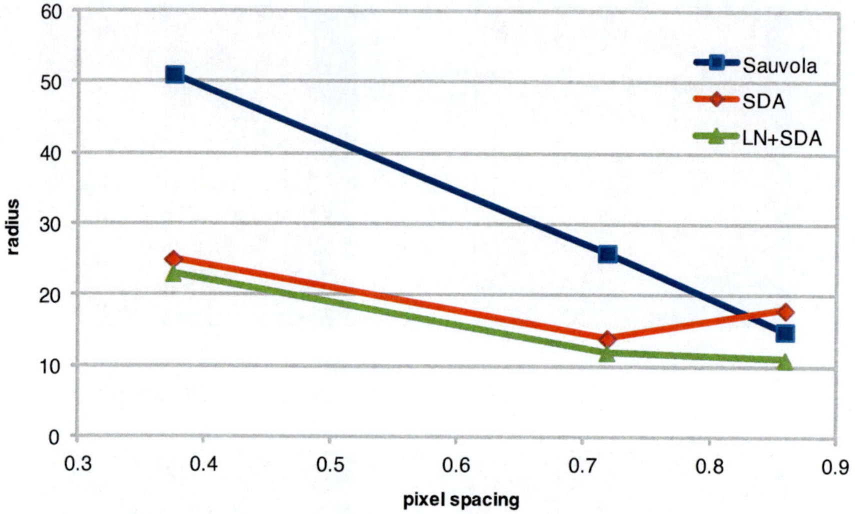

Fig. 7. Radius and pixel spacing relation.

4 Summary

The challenge of detecting such objects can be tackled by local approaches that focus on pixels and their neighborhoods. As shown by the results, the local averaging thresholds also did not produce satisfactory values. However, three algorithms turned out to be a good approach to this problem: Sauvola threshold, the Statistical Dominance Algorithm, and a combination of SDA and Local Normalization, which helps to emphasize lesions in images. Although high precision was achieved by two approaches (Sauvola and LN+SDA), these methods could not be used for fully automated plaque detection. Therefore, further investigations should be conducted.

Acknowledgements. This publication was funded by AGH University of Science and Technology, Faculty of Electrical Engineering, Automatics, Computer Science and Biomedical Engineering.

This work was co-financed by the AGH University of Science and Technology, Faculty of EAIIB, KBIB no 16.16.120.773.

References

1. Frey, B.M., Petersen, M., Mayer, C., Schulz, M., Cheng, B., Thomalla, G.: Characterization of white matter hyperintensities in large-scale MRI-studies. Front. Neurol. **10**, 238 (2019)
2. Oksuz, I.: Brain MRI artefact detection and correction using convolutional neural networks. Comput. Methods Prog. Biomed. **199**, 105909 (2020)

3. Kozub, J., Paciorek, A., Urbanik, A., Ostrogórska, M.: Effects of using different software packages for bold analysis in planning a neurosurgical treatment in patients with brain tumours. Clin. Imag. **68**, 148–157 (2020)
4. Naive: Nuclei counter. MATLAB Central File Exchange. https://www.mathworks.com/matlabcentral/fileexchange/45174-nuclei-counter
5. Zhao, M., et al.: Seens: nuclei segmentation in pap smear images with selective edge enhancement. Fut. Gen. Comput. Syst. **114**, 185–194 (2020)
6. Gertych, A., Ma, Z., Tajbakhsh, J., Velasquez-Vacca, A., Knudsen, B.S.: Rapid 3-D delineation of cell nuclei for high-content screening platforms. Comput. Biol. Med. **69**, 328–338 (2016)
7. Loy, G., Zelinsky, A.: Fast radial symmetry for detecting points of interest. IEEE Trans. Patt. Anal. Mach. Intell. **25**(8), 959–973 (2003)
8. Soille, P.: Morphological Image Analysis. Springer, Berlin (2004). https://doi.org/10.1007/978-3-662-05088-0
9. Bernsen, J.: Dynamic thresholding of gray-level images. In: Proceedings of the Eighth International Conference on Pattern Recognition, Paris (1986)
10. Sezgin, M., Sankur, B.: Survey over image thresholding techniques and quantitative performance evaluation. J. Electr. Imag. **13**(1), 146–166 (2004)
11. Otsu, N.: A threshold selection method from gray-level histograms. IEEE Trans, Syst. Man Cybernet. **9**(1), 62–66 (1979)
12. Niblack, W.: An Introduction to Digital Image Processing, pp. 115–116. Prentice Hall, Englewood Cliffs (1986)
13. Sauvola, J., Pietikäinen, M.: Adaptive document image binarization. Patt. Recogn. **33**(2), 225–236 (2000)
14. Phansalkar, N., More, S., Sabale, A., Joshi, M.: Adaptive local thresholding for detection of nuclei in diversity stained cytology images. In: 2011 International Conference on Communications and Signal Processing, pp. 218–220. IEEE (2011)
15. Piórkowski, A.: A Statistical dominance algorithm for edge detection and segmentation of medical images. In: Piętka, E., Badura, P., Kawa, J., Wieclawek, W. (eds.) Information Technologies in Medicine. AISC, vol. 471, pp. 3–14. Springer, Cham (2016). https://doi.org/10.1007/978-3-319-39796-2_1
16. Iwaszenko, S., Róg, L.: Coal images database and its application for selected coal grains properties analysis. In: IOP Conference Series: Materials Science and Engineering, vol. 545, p. 012003. IOP Publishing, Bristol (2019)
17. Nurzynska, K., Mikhalkin, A., Piorkowski, A.: CAS: cell annotation software - research on neuronal tissue has never been so transparent. Neuroinformatics **15**, 365–382 (2017)
18. Sage, D., Unser, M.: Easy Java programming for teaching image-processing. In: Proceedings 2001 International Conference on Image Processing, vol. 3, pp. 298–301. IEEE (2001)
19. Mutterer, J., Rasband, W.: Imagej macro language programmers reference guide v1. 46d. RSB Homepage, pp. 1–45 (2012)
20. Schneider, C.A., Rasband, W.S., Eliceiri, K.W.: NIH image to ImageJ: 25 years of image analysis. Nat. Methods **9**(7), 671–675 (2012)
21. Nichele, L., Persichetti, V., Lucidi, M., Cincotti, G.: Quantitative evaluation of ImageJ thresholding algorithms for microbial cell counting. OSA Contin. **3**(6), 1417–1427 (2020). https://doi.org/10.1364/OSAC.393971

Gastrointestinal Microbiome Changes Directly Connect to the Control of Behavioral Processes Which Could Be Verified by Means of a New Bioimpedance Measurement Technique

Kitti Mintál[1,2,3(✉)], Attila Tóth[1,2,3], Anita Kovács[1,2], Edina Hormay[1,2,3], Adorján Varga[4], Béla Kocsis[4], Zoltán Vizvári[3,5], László Lénárd[1,2,3], and Zoltán Karádi[1,2,3]

[1] Medical School, Institute of Physiology, University of Pécs, Pécs, Hungary
kitti.mintal@aok.pte.hu

[2] Medical School, Homeostatic Control Research Group, University of Pécs, Pécs, Hungary

[3] Cellular Bioimpedance Research Group, Szentágothai Research Centre, University of Pécs, Pécs, Hungary

[4] Medical School, Department of Medical Microbiology and Immunology, University of Pécs, Pécs, Hungary

[5] Department of Environmental Engineering, Faculty of Engineering and Information Technology, University of Pécs, Pécs, Hungary

Abstract. In recent years, our knowledge on the intestinal microbiota has greatly improved. Dysfunctions of the gut microbiome have been shown to cause alterations of peripheral and central regulatory processes, ultimately leading to functional deficits in brain functions, including those in behavior.

Therefore, the first aim of the present study was to generate alterations of the gut microbiome and to investigate these effects as well as those of the probiotic treatment on behavior. To do so, we divided adult male Wistar rats into four - 1. antibiotic treated; 2. antibiotic and probiotic treated; 3. probiotic treated; 4. control - groups. Behavioral tests were conducted following microbiota manipulations. To make sure that the antibiotic treatment has not caused changes of body composition which itself could influence the behavior, a new non-invasive body composition measurement technique was introduced.

The findings demonstrate significant group differences in the behavioral tests. By the bioimpedance technology, we did not observe serious body composition changes among the groups. These results confirm our hypothesis that antibiotic-induced gut dysbiosis directly influences the control of behavioral processes.

N. Piaseczna et al. (Eds.): EMBS ICS 2020, AISC 1360, pp. 106–109, 2022.
https://doi.org/10.1007/978-3-030-88976-0_14

Keywords: Brain-gut-microbiota axis · Gut microbiota · Bioimpedance

1 Introduction

It has been shown recently that disruptions in the composition of the gut ecology are with adverse consequences of homeostatic functions. Namely, the altered gut microbiome appears to affect functioning of the central nervous system, which results in such dysfunctions through the microbiome - brain - gut axis [1,2]. Alterations of the gut microbiota can be caused by numerous factors, and the worldwide increasing consumption of antibiotics certainly represents one of these. The expanded consumption of antibiotics is recently considered to be involved in the development of autism spectrum disorders. To substantiate this hypothesis, we employed an antibiotic animal model to explore the effects of gut microbiome depletion (gut dysbiosis) on cognitive processes [3]. In addition, we also aimed to investigate its potency to modify other alterations of the gut microbiome on emotional, cognitive and social behavioral responses.

2 Methods

We used adult male Wistar rats. Animals have been divided into four groups:

1. antibiotic (broad spectrum antibiotic mixture for 4 weeks) treated;
2. antibiotic and probiotic treated;
3. probiotic treated;
4. control ones.

Substances were dissolved in the animals' drinking water. The probiotic mixture (beneficial bacterial species) was given right after the antibiotic treatment and the third group received only probiotic mix for 14 days. Behavioral tests (open field, 3 chamber social, and passive avoidance tests, respectively) were carried out following the treatments.

3 Results

These behavioral tests verified significant group differences. Antibiotic treated rats spent significantly less time in the central zone and the number of abandoned pellets was also higher among them than in rats of the other groups; all these results seem to indicate depression-like behavior (see Fig. 1). This behavior, however, was no longer noticed after the probiotic treatment. Spending shorter time in the corners also confirms the postulation that the probiotic could attenuate depression-like behavior. We also carried out a social interaction test which has shown antisocial behavior among the antibiotic treated rats.

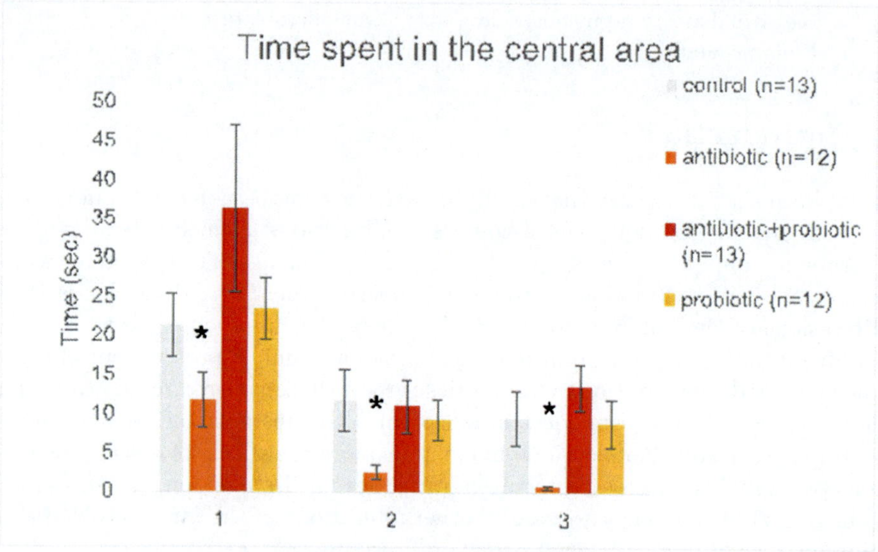

Fig. 1. Altered behavior following antibiotic treatment.

Nevertheless, to exclude that the antibiotic treatment induced discomfort was due to changes of body composition which itself could influence the behavior, we introduced a new electrical impedance spectrum analysis based, non-invasive body composition measurement technique. Our research group developed a four-electrode ultra-low frequency bioimpedance measurement technology, which enabled us to perform high-precision full-body composition measurements. By means of these experiments, we could verify that gut microbiome alterations can change the behavior without changing body composition.

4 Conclusion

As predicted, alterations of the microbiota appeared to play an important modulating role in the central regulatory processes. The findings demonstrated that our probiotic mixture improve gut microbiota conditions, attenuating depression-like behavior. By the bioimpedance technique, no significant body composition differences were found among the groups. Thus, our data substantiated that antibiotic-induced gut dysbiosis - without body composition alterations - directly influences the control of behavioral processes.

References

1. Sampson, T.R., Mazmanian, S.K.: Control of brain development, function, and behavior by the microbiome. Cell Host Microbe. **17**, 565–576 (2015)

2. Martin, C.R., Osadchiy, V., Kalani, A., Mayer, E.A.: The brain-gut-microbiome axis. Cell Mol Gastroenterol. Hepatol. **6**, 133–148 (2018)
3. Fröhlich, E.E., et al.: Cognitive impairment by antibiotic-induced gut dysbiosis: analysis of gut microbiota-brain communication. Brain Behav. Immun. **56**, 140–55 (2016)

Scatter Comparison of Heart Rate Variability Parameters

Antonina Pater[1,2](✉) and Mateusz Soliński[1]

[1] Faculty of Physics, Warsaw University of Technology, Warsaw, Poland
[2] Nałęcz Institute of Biocybernetics and Biomedical Engineering, Polish Academy of Sciences, Warsaw, Poland
apater@ibib.waw.pl

Abstract. Heart rate variability (HRV) is a simple and non-invasive method for autonomous nervous system activity and probability of cardiovascular morbidity and mortality monitoring. However, the high scatter of HRV parameter values, found in both intraindividual and homogeneous intergroup measurements, inhibits the process of determining normal values or the ones indicating certain diseases. Such a process could be useful in clinical practice.

The aim of this work was to compare the scatter of a selection of HRV parameters from linear, frequency and nonlinear domains. They were compared using three different methods: between persons, between consecutive nights and between 45 min fragments of RR time intervals.

The largest mean scatter of HRV parameters was found in method 2 and the lowest in method 1. In all scales, correlation dimension, Lyapunov exponent, and unnormalized frequency parameters were the most scattered among the methods. Shannon entropy, Hurst exponent, DFA method's α exponent and mean RR interval had the lowest scatter. Low scatter of HRV parameters may be useful for determining the normal values of a parameter, however the quality of information carried by HRV parameter should be considered too.

The questionnaire revealed that the subjects formed a uniform group regarding the daytime events. Most participants did not have any highly stressful or exciting events. The sleep quality, however, was distributed almost equally over the possible answers.

The large dispersion of most parameters in different time scales indicates a high uncertainty in the interpretation of single measurements of the series of RR time intervals, because they may deviate from the typical values for the patient. The allostatic regulation of the organism should be considered using the averaged results to minimize the impact of intraindividual and interindividual variability.

Keywords: Heart rate variability · Autonomous nervous system · Nonlinear methods · Repeatability

N. Piaseczna et al. (Eds.): EMBS ICS 2020, AISC 1360, pp. 110–117, 2022.
https://doi.org/10.1007/978-3-030-88976-0_15

1 Introduction

Heart rate variability (HRV) is recognized as a measure of autonomous nervous system activity. Moreover, it is also used for prediction of cardiovascular diseases and their development, including the risk of sudden cardiac death [1]. However normal values or intervals characteristic for cardiovascular diseases are missing. One of the reasons behind that state is a high scatter of parameter values found in both intraindividual and intergroup measurements [2].

The aim of the study is an analysis of the variability of night-time heart rhythm recordings obtained from healthy subjects during 7 days long observation of daily activity and a comparison of repeatability of 27 different method of HRV analysis available in literature. Since there is no publicly available dataset containing seven consecutive night-time RR interval series nor ECG recordings, during the study such measurements were carried out.

2 Materials and Methods

2.1 Data

Fourteen volunteers, of which 8 were men participated in the study. Their mean age was 23.3(2.0) years. In the beginning they were instructed how to use a Holter device and to avoid coffee and alcohol for at least 8 h before sleep. Then, for seven consecutive nights they were carrying out measurements using three-lead Holter ECG device (Lifecard CF, Spacelabs Healthcare). Each recording was made during subjects' sleep and had to be at least seven hour long.

Additionally, participants wore Fitbit bands and filled in questionnaires to ensure similar conditions, such as whether any heavily emotional events occurred.

The ECG recordings were processed using Sentinel by Spacelabs Healthcare. The program was used to annotate R waves and to extract a series of RR time intervals for further analysis.

RR intervals series were then cut to 6 h long excerpts to remove the time spent on falling asleep and waking up.

RR intervals representing ectopic beats were withdrawn from analysis. Before frequency analysis, RR time series were resampled 1 Hz.

2.2 Analysis of HRV Derived Parameters

Time and frequency domain HRV parameters used in the study are presented in Table 1. A wider discussion of these measures can be found in [1].

In Table 2 nonlinear domain HRV parameters used in the study are shown.

The HRV parameters were compared using three different approaches: on a subject basis (method 1), on a night basis (method 2), and on a 45-min long fragments basis (method 3). The three methods are described in the following:

Method 1: Scatter comparison between subjects
Method scheme:

Table 1. Time and frequency domain measures of HRV.

Short name	Description	Domain
Mean RR	Mean length of all RR interval	Time
SDNN	Standard deviation of all RR intervals	Time
RMSS	The square root of the mean of the sum of the squares of differences between adjacent RR intervals	Time
pNN50	Number of pairs of adjacent NN intervals differing by more than 50 ms in the entire recording divided by the total number of all NN intervals	Time
HF	Power in high frequency range (0.15–0.4 Hz)	Frequency
LF	Power in low frequency range (0.04–0.15 Hz)	Frequency
VLF	Power in very low frequency range (0.04 Hz)	Frequency
HFnorm	HF/(HF+LF)	Frequency
LFnorm	LF/(HF+LF)	Frequency

Table 2. Nonlinear domain measures of HRV.

Short names	Method name	Source
0 V, 1 V, 2 V	Porta's symbolic analysis	[3]
$\alpha 1, \alpha 2$	Detrended fluctuations analysis	[4]
S	Shannon entropy	[5]
SampEn	Sample entropy	[6]
H	Mean Hurst exponent from multiscale multifractal analysis	[7]
D2	Correlation dimension	[8]
L	Lyapunov exponent	[9]
SD1, SD2	Poincaré parameters	[10]
PIP, IALS, PPS, PAS	Fragmentation parameters	[11]

1. Calculation of HRV parameters for each RR series
2. Calculation of mean values of all 7 nights for each subject
3. Calculation of percentage difference of each mean value from point 2 and global mean (mean of all subjects' mean values).

Method 2: Scatter comparison between nights
Method scheme:

1. Calculation of HRV parameters for each RR series
2. Calculation of percentage difference of each value from point 1 and global mean.

Method 3: Scatter comparison between 45 min fragments
Method scheme:

1. Each RR series is divided into 8 parts (6h/8 = 45 min).
2. Calculation of HRV parameters for each fragment.
3. Calculation of mean values for each subject.
4. Calculation of percentage difference of each of mean values from point 3 and global mean (mean of given subject's mean values).

For each method and parameter, the mean value and standard deviation were calculated.

3 Results

Figures 1, 2, 3 show the boxplots with percentage differences of parameters for each scatter comparison method. The boxplots are ordered by the mean value of the difference. In the first method, 14 measurement points were obtained; in method 2:95 measurement points (that is, 14 subjects times 7 nights and 3 nights excluded from analysis) and in method 3: 760 measurement points (that is 14 subjects times 7 nights – 3 nights excluded and all that times 8 parts). Mean values calculated for each of the scatter comparison methods are shown in Table 3.

Table 3. Mean percentage differences of parameters calculated for each method. Method 1 – scatter be-tween subjects, method 2 – nights, method 3 – 45 min fragments.

Parameter	Method 1 [%] (n = 14)	Method 2 [%] (n = 95)	Method 3 [%] (n = 760)
meanRR	9.1(59)	9.8(6.6)	4,9(3.9)
SDNN	18(18)	20(18)	18(14)
pNN50	33(30)	38(28)	28(29)
RMSSD	29(33)	31(33)	18(14)
Shannon	5.3(4.8)	5.8(5.1)	6.6(5.1)
SampEn	10.9(8.5)	17(12)	17(15)
SD1	32(33)	34(38)	19(16)
SD2	18(16)	19(17)	19(14)
V0	22(19)	26(21)	26(24)
V1	16(14)	22(18)	16(13)
V2	30(36)	38(41)	27(23)
VLF	47(41)	48(43)	44(34)
LF	37(26)	39(29)	38(31)
HF	63(93)	68(93)	34(30)
TF	44(48)	46(48)	35(27)
HFnorm	20(16)	22(15)	15(12)
LFnorm	19(15)	21(14)	16(15)
PIP	11.2(8.0)	12.5(8.4)	7.8(6.6)
IALS	19(13)	22(14)	14(13)
PPS	10.6(8.6)	12.1(9.4)	11.4(9.7)
PAS	17(11)	19(12)	15(13)
alphaT	3.3(2.6)	4.6(3.0)	6.9(6.1)

For the majority of the parameters, the lowest scatter was found in method 1 (the one measuring scatter between subjects). The highest scatter was observed in method 2 (scatter between nights). Percentage differences from method 3 have similar values to method 1 and in case of 12 parameters they have higher values than method 1.

Lyapunov exponent L and correlation dimension D2 have large percentage difference values of scatter in all comparison methods. Other parameters with high scatter are frequency parameters (VLF, LF, HF, TF), but their normed forms have significantly lower scatter.

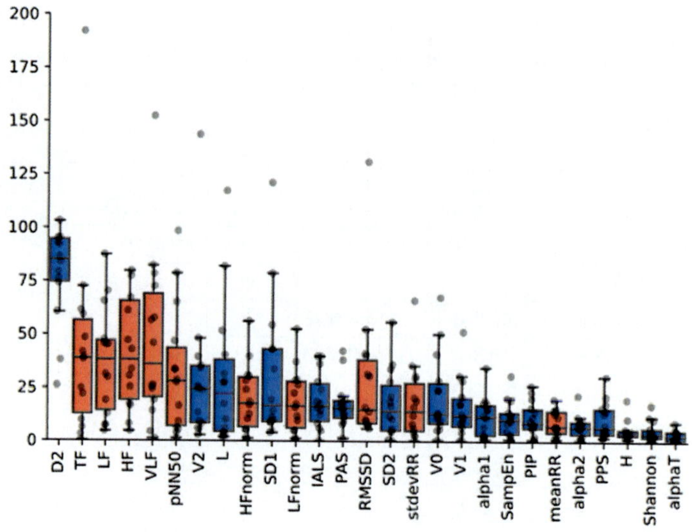

Fig. 1. Scatter of parameters in method 1 - scatter comparison between subjects. Non-linear methods shown in blue.

For each RR interval series, Hurst surfaces were calculated using Multiscale Multifractal Analysis. Changes of the shapes of the surfaces between consecutive nights were observed.

One subject was found to have supraventricular ectopic beats of the order of a few hundred per night. Nevertheless, the subjects considered themselves to be healthy.

Pearson correlation factor was calculated between pairs of percentage differences of values from each method. The highest number of correlation factors greater than 0.5 was found in method 2. Additionally, for the two most distinct methods (1 and 3), differences in Pearson factor values were measured. There were 10 pairs with a difference higher than 0.8.

The questionnaire revealed that the subjects formed a uniform group regarding the daytime events. Most participants did not have any highly stressful or exciting events. The sleep quality, however, was distributed almost equally over the possible answers.

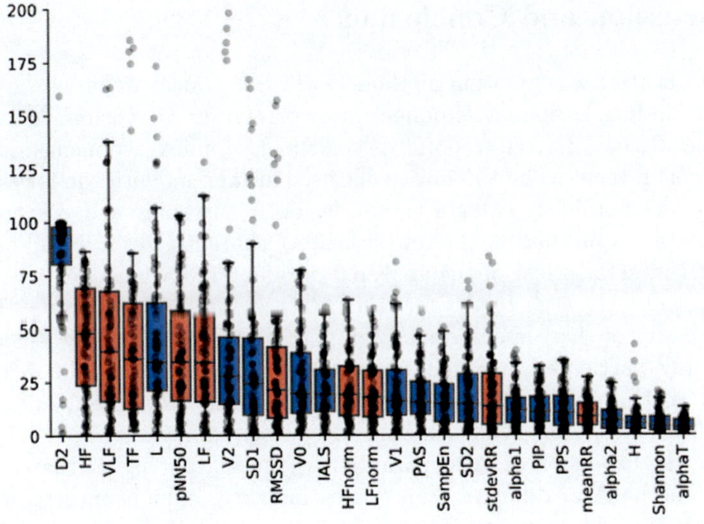

Fig. 2. Scatter of parameters in method 2 - scatter comparison between nights. Non-linear methods shown in blue.

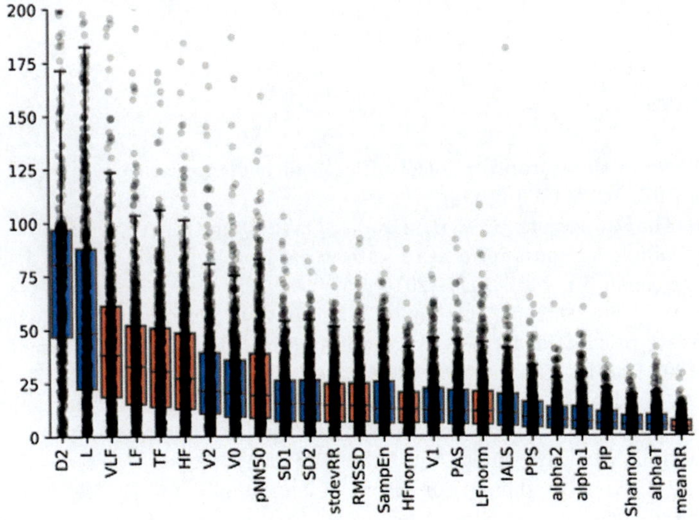

Fig. 3. Scatter of parameters in method 3 - scatter comparison between nights. Non-linear methods shown in blue.

4 Discussion and Conclusion

The lowest scatter was found in method 1, which is a measure of intergroup variability. Excluding Lyapunov exponent and correlation dimension, scatter range was from 3.3(2.6)% for αT to 63(93)% for HF. Lyapunov exponent and correlation dimension seem to be the most volatile. Parameters with the lowest scatter belong to the nonlinear category, that is, both entropies and αT coefficient. Exceptionally, in method 3, the lowest scatter characterizes a linear parameter - mean RR interval. Most of the analyzed parameters have similar scatter in all methods.

The quality of the presented research may be compromised by the low number of study participants. Higher number of participants should increase the reliability of the results. It may be useful to consider adding a questionnaire designed by a sleep quality specialist or by a sleep laboratory.

The large dispersion of most parameters (the scatter higher than 20% in at least one method) in different time scales indicates a high uncertainty in the interpretation of single measurements of the series of RR time intervals, because they may deviate from the typical values of the patient. Taking into account the allostatic regulation of the organism, the use of the averaged results should be considered to minimize the impact of intraindividual and interindividual variability.

References

1. Task Force of the European Society Electrophysiology: Heart rate variability. Circulation **93**, 1043–1065 (1996)
2. Nunan, D., Sandercock, G.R.H., Brodie, D.A.: Quantitative systematic review of normal values for short-term heart rate variability in healthy adults. Pacing Clin. Electrophysiol. **33**, 1407–1417 (2010)
3. Porta, A., et al.: Entropy, entropy rate, and pattern classification as tools to typify complexity in short heart period variability series. IEEE Trans. Biomed. Eng. **48**, 1282–1291 (2001)
4. Peng, C.-K., Havlin, S., Stanley, H.E., Goldberger, A.L.: Quantification of scaling exponents and crossover phenomena in nonstationary heartbeat time series. Chaos Interdisciplinary J. Nonlinear Sci. **5**, 82–87 (1995)
5. Shannon, C.E.: A mathematical theory of communication. Bell Syst. Tech. J. **27**, 379–423 (1948)
6. Richman, J.S., Moorman, J.R.: Physiological time-series analysis using approximate entropy and sample entropy. Am. J. Physiol. Heart Circulatory Physiol. **278**, H2039–H2049 (2000)
7. Gierałtowski, J., Żebrowski, J.J., Baranowski, R.: Multiscale multifractal analysis of heart rate variability recordings with a large number of occurrences of arrhythmia. Phys. Rev. E **85**, 021925 (2012)
8. Grassberger, P., Procaccia, I.: Measuring the strangeness of strange attractors. In: Hunt, B.R., Li, T.Y., Kennedy, J.A., Nusse, H.E. (eds.) The Theory of Chaotic Attractors, pp. 170–189. Springer, New York (2004). https://doi.org/10.1007/978-0-387-21830-4_12

9. Rosenstein, M.T., Collins, J.J., Luca, C.J.D.: A practical method for calculating largest Lyapunov exponents from small data sets. Physica D Nonlinear Phenom. **65**, 117–134 (1993)
10. Golińska, A.K.: Poincaré plots in analysis of selected biomedical signals. Stud. Logic Grammar Rhetoric **35**, 117–127 (2013)
11. Costa, M.D., Davis, R.B., Goldberger, A.L.: Heart rate fragmentation: a new approach to the analysis of cardiac interbeat interval dynamics. Front. Physiol. **8**, 255 (2017)

Automated External Contour-Segmentation Method for Vertebrae in Lateral Cervical Spine Radiographs

Zofia Schneider(✉) and Elżbieta Pociask

BioMedical Imaging Science Club, Department of Biocybernetics and Biomedical Engineering, AGH University of Science and Technology, Krakow, Poland
schneider@student.agh.edu.pl

Abstract. Spondyloarthritis (SpA) is a group of inflammatory diseases that cause severe damage in the structure of the skeleton. One of the most important features that are assessed in the diagnosis of SpA disorders and during the monitoring of the progression of this disease is the shape of the vertebrae and the appearance of bony outgrowths in the spine region. For this purpose, radiography is often used. This paper presents a novel automated method of external contour segmentation of vertebrae in X-ray images. The proposed algorithm consists of preprocessing, edge detection using the Sobel operator, binarization, area opening, and skeletonization. During the study, the impact of different filters (i.e., Gaussian filter, sigma filter, and anisotropic diffusion filter) on the quality of the results was also investigated. The method's efficiency was tested on a dataset containing 11 lateral cervical spine radiographs. The results show that the method has the potential to become an automatic tool used by physicians to determine the shape of vertebrae.

Keywords: Image processing · X-ray · Radiograph · Vertebrae · Spondyloarthritis · Bone segmentation · Edge detection

1 Introduction

1.1 Clinical Importance and Motivation

X-raying is one of the most commonly used medical imaging techniques, especially in the diagnosis of bone diseases or injuries. Radiographs provide a lot of information about anatomical structures and other objects. One feature that can be assessed with the use of this imaging technique is the shape of the bones, which is important, for instance, in the diagnosis of spondyloarthritis (SpA). This term refers to a group of inflammatory disorders which can cause severe damage in the spine structure. One SpA disease is ankylosing spondylitis. This disorder starts with chronic inflammation of intravertebral ligaments and joints

N. Piaseczna et al. (Eds.): EMBS ICS 2020, AISC 1360, pp. 118–126, 2022.
https://doi.org/10.1007/978-3-030-88976-0_16

and subsequently leads to the formation of two types of bony outgrowths called osteophytes and syndesmophytes. As bone formation progresses, the syndesmophytes grow together with the adjacent vertebrae, leading to spinal stiffness and a major decrease of the patient's mobility [1,2]. Ankylosing spondylitis can progress quickly and cause serious damage. Therefore, early diagnosis and monitoring of the shape of the vertebrae are crucial if therapy is to be effective. In order to improve the healing process, it is essential to understand the behavior and flexibility of the vertebral connections. Magnetic resonance is usually used to assess inflammation, which is strongly related to the progression of SpA diseases; however, radiography and computer tomography (CT) are mostly used to monitor vertebrae shape and the presence of syndesmophytes.

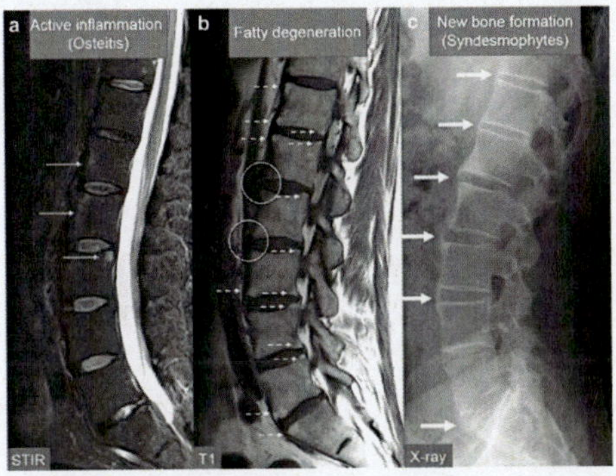

Fig. 1. MRI and X-ray images of the spine of a patient suffering from SpA. The MRI scans show active inflammation (a) and fatty degeneration (b), while syndesmophytes are also clearly visible in the radiograph (c) [3]

To improve the diagnosis and monitoring of the progression of SpA diseases, there is a need to develop an automatic tool that could be used by physicians in daily clinical practice to determine vertebrae shape in X-ray images.

1.2 State of the Art

Over the years, many methodologies and computer-assisted quantitative tools have been intensively developed to analyze radiographs and extract features of the objects present in them. The literature mainly recommends edge-based segmentation techniques [4], but these are not the only methods that can be used. The bones of the hand and wrist are segmented using, for instance, region growing and merging [5], or top-hat transform and fractal analysis [6]. The method of bone segmentation which was proposed in [7] uses multi-scale Canny edge detection and histogram analysis. Thresholding and analysis of contour maps are used to segment the bones of the hand in X-ray images in [8]. The algorithm proposed in [9] uses connected-component labeling for segmentation of teeth from digitized dental radiographic films. Most studies in this field focus on the segmentation of the hand, wrist, and arm bones in X-ray images or teeth in panoramic radiographs. Vertebrae segmentation is not a well-researched issue, but some approaches to this subject have also been proposed in the literature. These algorithms are based on, for example, the Active Appearance Model [10], the Hough Transform [11] or Partial Shape Matching [12]. Mostly, these methods provide satisfying results, but they still require human input, e.g. selection of the region of interest (ROI) or manual setting of filter parameters.

The aim of this paper is to propose an automatic method of extracting the shape of vertebrae from radiographs using morphological operations and classical edge detectors.

This paper is organized in 5 sections as follows. Section 1 presents the motivation for our work and a review of the state of the art in radiograph processing. Section 2 describes an overview of the implemented algorithm. In Sects. 3 and 4, the conducted tests and results are described. Section 5 closes the paper with conclusions, a discussion of the results, and possible future directions for research.

2 Materials and Methods

The first part presents in detail the technical and medical aspects of spine radiographs. Data were collected from 11 patients at the University Hospital in Krakow, Poland; this data was anonymized [13]. In the second part, we concentrate on the proposed algorithm and its particular steps. The flowchart of the proposed algorithm is illustrated in Fig. 2.

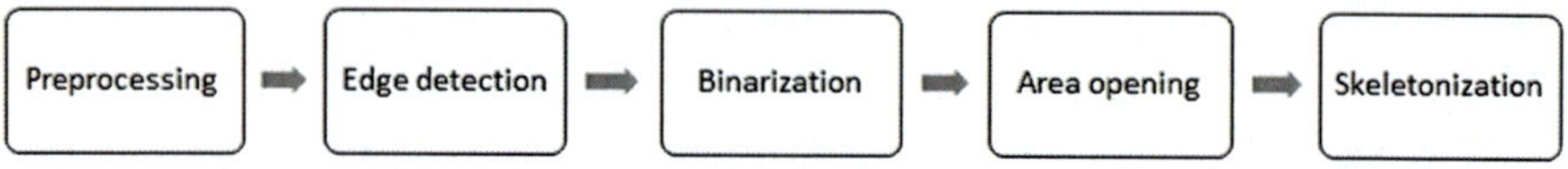

Fig. 2. Flowchart of the proposed algorithm.

2.1 Radiographs

The algorithm's performance was tested on 11 lateral cervical spine radiographs [14]. All the images are in PNG format with a color depth of 8 bits. The radiographs are of different quality and lightness, as can be seen in Fig. 3; some of them contain significant noise. Therefore, preprocessing was a crucial step in the analysis of the data.

For each radiograph, the dataset also contains an image whose edges have been detected. These contours were obtained semi-automatically under the supervision of a radiologist and they were used as a reference in the results validation of this study. The ImageJ environment (version 1.53c) was used for image processing.

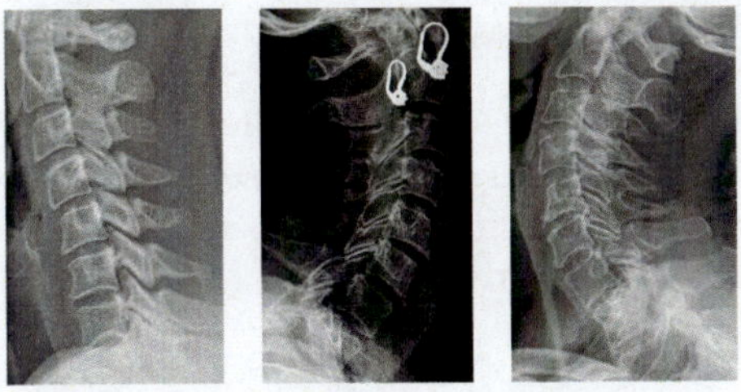

Fig. 3. Sample images from the dataset.

2.2 Radiographs Preprocessing

Preprocessing is realized in two steps. The first stage is denoising. To find the optimal preprocessing method, different filters were tested: Gaussian blur, Sigma filter and anisotropic diffusion filter.

Gaussian smoothing is a denoising technique which uses the Gaussian function to calculate the coefficients of the kernel, which is then used to convolve the image. The resulting image is blurred, and the smoothing intensity depends on the size of the kernel and the value of the standard deviation σ [15].

The second preprocessing smoothing technique which was tested was a sigma filter. In this method, the value of each pixel is replaced with the average intensity of its neighbors; however, the only neighbors that are considered are those whose intensity lies within a given number of standard deviations (sigmas) from the current pixel's value [16]. The sigma filter plugin in ImageJ has three parameters which impact the smoothing effect: window radius, i.e. number of pixels taken as neighbors; the number of sigmas; and the minimum pixel fraction.

Anisotropic diffusion, which is the third tested filter, is a more complicated preprocessing method. It uses a Gaussian filter to smooth the image but reduces the diffusivity in parts of the image which have a high likelihood of being edges. To calculate the likelihood, gradient and divergency are used. Anisotropic diffusion is performed iteratively: the diffusion equation is applied to the image that was obtained in the previous iteration. This process is repeated a set number of times [17].

The next preprocessing stage is contrast enhancement, which is performed using Contrast Limited Adaptive Histogram Equalization (CLAHE). With this method, the histogram is not equalized globally for the whole image; instead, a separate histogram is computed for the neighborhood of each pixel. To avoid amplifying the noise in homogeneous areas where there is a high histogram peak, contrast limitation is implemented by clipping the histogram to a predefined value and redistributing the clipped pixels uniformly to other histogram bins. Only after this operation is the histogram equalized [18]. When using CLAHE, three parameters can be manipulated: the block size, i.e., the size of a local region for which the histogram is equalized; the number of histogram bins used for its equalization; and the maximum slope, which limits the contrast stretch.

2.3 Radiograph Segmentation

Edge Detection. In the proposed method, the edges in the image are detected using the Sobel operator. The image is convolved with two 3×3 kernels to obtain sharp vertical and horizontal intensity changes. The result is the square root of the sum of the squares of the derivatives [19].

Binarization. The next stage of the algorithm is binarization, which is performed using thresholding. The threshold is set automatically by the isodata algorithm. With this method, the threshold value is iteratively searched for until it is at the same distance from the average intensity of the pixels below and above the threshold [20].

Area Opening. After binarization, the area-opening operation is performed, which consists in removing from the binary image objects whose area is smaller than the preset number of pixels [21]. Some X-ray images may be very noisy, in which case the initial filtering may not be sufficient. In this case, after thresholding, there may be a lot of small objects in the image which are caused by noise and are not part of the vertebrae contours. The aim of this stage is to eliminate these objects.

Skeletonization. The final image is obtained by skeletonizing the result of the previous steps. This operation consists in iteratively removing pixels from the edges of objects until they are reduced to one-pixel-wide contours [22].

3 Statistical Analysis

During the analysis of the obtained results, it was noticed that the contours were often shifted by 1 or 2 pixels compared to the reference outlines. Thus, statistical analysis of the algorithm's efficiency was performed by calculating the accuracy with 1, 2, and 3 pixels. To compute this parameter, the reference outlines were dilated using structuring elements (SE) with different radii (r = 0, 1, 2, 3 pixels). The contours obtained using the proposed method were then compared with each dilation result. The accuracy was calculated as the percentage of pixels of the resulting contour that were overlapped by the unchanged and dilated reference contours. The calculations were performed according to the equation:

$$x = \frac{N_1}{N_2} \cdot 100\%, \qquad (1)$$

where N1 is the number of pixels whose value in both compared images is 1, and N2 is the number of pixels of the resulting outline. A graphical presentation of this validation method can be seen in Fig. 4.

In order to complete the evaluation, calculations were also performed conversely: the percentage of pixels of the reference outline that were overlapped by the dilated result of the proposed algorithm was calculated. Although both the reference and the resulting images contained the edges of all the objects in the radiographs, they were compared only in the region of interest, i.e., external vertebra contours.

4 Results and Discussion

The parameters described in the previous section were calculated for all 11 images in the dataset. The results are presented in Tables 1 and 2. The outlines for which the evaluation was performed were obtained using a Gaussian filter ($\sigma = 2$) and CLAHE (block size = 200, histogram bins = 256, maximum slope = 3) as preprocessing.

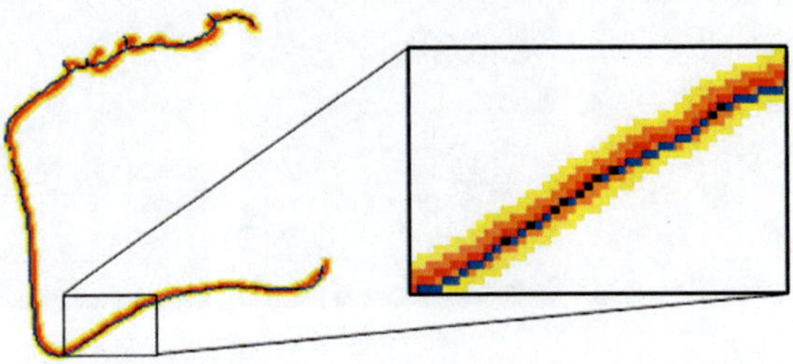

Fig. 4. Graphical evaluation of segmentation accuracy for a single sample vertebra with a zoomed view of a fragment. Color key: red line – reference contour; blue line – contour obtained using the proposed method; black line – overlap of the reference and obtained contours; orange line – reference contour dilated with SE radius of 1; yellow line – reference contour dilated with SE radius of 2.

Table 1. Percentage of the outline's pixels obtained using the proposed method that were overlapped by the reference outline, which was dilated by SE of radius r

	r = 0	r = 1	r = 2	r = 3
Mean	26.74	71.38	87.27	94.21
Median	28.12	73.92	89.17	95.63
Standard deviation	4.92	6.32	4.15	2.68

Table 2. Percentage of the reference outline's pixels that were overlapped by the outline that was obtained using the proposed method and dilated by SE of radius r

	r = 0	r = 1	r = 2	r = 3
Mean	21.57	61.46	75.38	81.46
Median	21.53	60.65	75.50	81.08
Standard deviation	2.88	5.57	4.61	4.02

As mentioned previously, the resulting outlines were slightly shifted. Therefore, the average accuracy when the raw outlines without dilation are compared amounts only to 26.74%; however, it increases to 71.38% after dilation of the reference outline using SE with a radius of 1 pixel, and it increases to 94.21% for an SE radius of 3. The second parameter shows that even if the outlines were shifted, most of the vertebrae edges were detected.

Figure 5 shows the results obtained using different preprocessing techniques: Gaussian filter, sigma filter, and anisotropic diffusion filter. It can be clearly seen that preprocessing is a crucial stage because the outline obtained without using any filter is noisy and full of artifacts, which makes it unsatisfactory. However, it seems that all of the tested filters fulfill their function and work similarly on all the images from the dataset. Nevertheless, the performance of the filters highly depends on the values of their parameters, so more thorough research should be performed on this subject to find the optimal preprocessing technique for the algorithm. Such an investigation is planned by the authors of this paper.

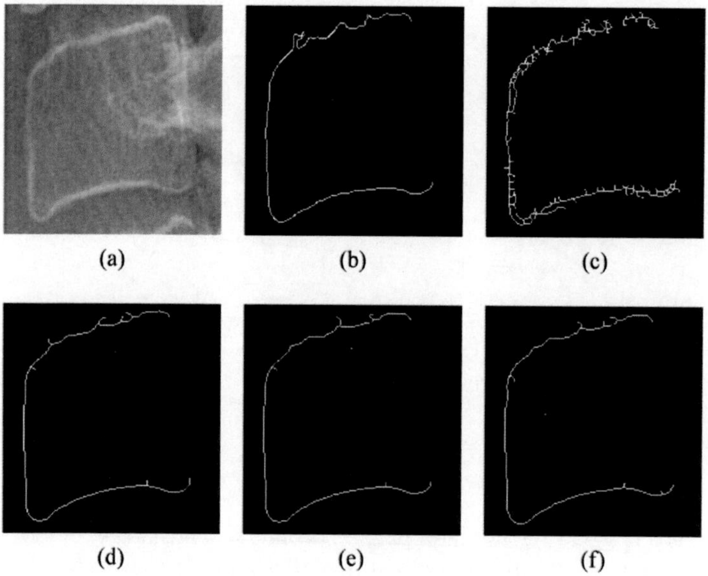

Fig. 5. Comparison of results obtained using different preprocessing techniques: a) original image; b) reference outline; c) without preprocessing; d) Gaussian filter (σ = 2); e) sigma filter (σ = 3, number of pixels = 3, minimum pixel fraction = 0.01); f) anisotropic diffusion filter (iterations = 7, smoothings per iteration = 1, edge threshold height = 20).

5 Conclusion and Future Plans

This study shows the potential role of a novel algorithm which could become a tool used by radiologists to determine the shape of vertebrae. Moreover, the method is fully automatic, therefore it does not need any human interference, unlike most existing techniques. However, the study is in its initial phase and the authors plan to develop the algorithm and improve its efficiency and accuracy. Firstly, the algorithm should be tested on another dataset to examine its performance under different conditions. As mentioned previously, the impact of the preprocessing filter and its parameters on the results will be examined more thoroughly. The quality of the segmentation results could also be improved in order to eliminate pixel bias and artifacts and discontinuities in the outlines. Nevertheless, although the outlines are not flawless, in most cases the vertebra shape was successfully captured, which was the main purpose of the algorithm.

Conflict of Interest

This publication was co-funded by AGH University of Science and Technology, Faculty of Electrical Engineering, Automatics, Computer Science and Biomedical Engineering under grant number 16.16.120.773. The authors declare that there is no conflict of interests regarding the publication of this paper.

References

1. Zimmermann-Górska, I.: Choroby reumatyczne. PZWL, Warszawa, pp. 35–37 (1989)
2. Zimmermann-Góska, I.: Reumatologia kliniczna. PZWL, Warszawa, vol. 2, pp. 729–741 (2008)
3. Poddubnyy, D., Sieper, J.: Mechanism of new bone formation in axial spondyloarthritis. Curr. Rheumatol. Rep **19**(9), 1–9 (2017). https://doi.org/10.1007/s11926-017-0681-5
4. Lee, L.K., Liew, S.C., Thong, W.J.: A review of image segmentation methodologies in medical image. In: Sulaiman, H.A., Othman, M.A., Othman, M.F.I., Rahim, Y.A., Pee, N.C. (eds.) Advanced Computer and Communication Engineering Technology. LNEE, vol. 315, pp. 1069–1080. Springer, Cham (2015). https://doi.org/10.1007/978-3-319-07674-4_99
5. Manos, G., Cairns, A., Ricketts, I., Sinclair, D.: Automatic segmentation of hand-wrist radi-ographs. Image Vis. Comput. **11**(2), 100–111 (1993)
6. Anam, S., Uchino, E., Suetake, N.: Hand bones radiograph segmentation by using novel method based on morphology and fractal. In: Joint 7th International Conference on Soft Computing and Intelligent Systems (SCIS) and 15th International Symposium on Advanced Intelligent Systems (ISIS), Kitakyushu, pp. 855–806 (2014)
7. Kazeminial, S., Karimil, N., Mirmahboub, B., Soroushmehr, S.M.R., Samavi, K., Najarian, K. Bone extraction in X-ray images by analysis of line fluctuations. In: IEEE International Conference on Image Preprocessing (ICIP), Quebec City, pp. 882–886 (2015)
8. Kuang-Yi, C., Chien-Sheng, L., Chin-Hsiang, C., Jen-Shiun, C., Chih-Hsien, H.: Using statistical parametric contour and threshold segmentation technology applied in X-ray bone images. In: International Symposium on Intelligent Signal Processing and Communication Systems (ISPACS), Phuket, pp. 1–5 (2016)
9. Said, E.H., Nassar, D.E.M., Fahmy, G., Ammar, H.H.: Teeth segmentation in digitized dental X-ray films using mathematical morphology. IEEE Trans. Inf. Forensics Secur. **1**(2), 178–189 (2006)

10. Nurzynska, K., et al.: Automatical syndesmophyte contour extraction from lateral c spine radio-graphs. In: Polish Conference on Biocybernetics and Biomedical Engineering, vol. 13, no. 10, pp. 164–173 (2017)
11. Zamora, G., Sari-Sarraf, H., Long, L.R.: Hierarchical segmentation of vertebrae from x-ray images. In: Medical Imaging: Image Processing, pp. 631–642 (2003)
12. Xu, X., Lee, D., Antani, S., Long, L.R.: A spine X-ray image retrieval system using partial shape matching. IEEE Trans. Inf. Technol. Biomed. **12**(1), 100–108 (2008)
13. Bielecka, M., Obuchowicz, R., Korkosz, M.: The shape language in application to the diagnosis of cervical vertebrae pathology. PLoS One **13**(10), e0204546 (2018)
14. Bielecka, M.: X-Ray spine images. OSF (2018)
15. Getreuer, P.: A survey of Gaussian convolution algorithms. Image Process. On Line **3**, 286–310 (2013)
16. Lee, J.S.: Digital image smoothing and the sigma filter. Comput. Vis. Graph. Image Process. **24**(2), 255–269 (1983)
17. Acton, S.T.: Diffusion partial differential equations for edge detection. In: The Essential Guide to Image Processing, pp. 525–552 (2009)
18. Zuiderveld, K.: Contrast Limited Adaptive Histogram Equalization. Graphics Gems, pp. 474–485 (1994)
19. Shrivakshan, G.T., Chandrasekar, C.: A comparison of various edge detection techniques used in image processing. IJCSI Int. J. Comput. Sci. Issues **9**(5), 269 (2012)
20. Zheng, C., Sun, D.W.: Image segmentation techniques. In: Computer Vision Technology for Food Quality Evaluation, pp. 37–56 (2008)
21. Vincent, L.: Morphological area openings and closings for grey-scale images. In: O, Y.L., Toet, A., Foster, D., Heijmans, H.J.A.M., Meer, P. (eds.) Shape in Picture. NATO ASI Series, vol. 126, pp. 197–208. Springer, Heidelberg (1994). https://doi.org/10.1007/978-3-662-03039-4_13
22. Zhang, T.Y., Suen, C.Y.: A fast parallel algorithm for thinning digital patterns. Commun. ACM **27**(3), 236–239 (1984)

Segmentation of a First Generation Agent Bubbles in the B-Mode Echocardiographic Images

Joanna Sorysz[1(✉)], Danuta Sorysz[2], and Adam Piórkowski[1]

[1] Department of Biocybernetics and Biomedical Engineering, AGH University of Science and Technology, Mickiewicza 30 Avenue, 30-059 Kraków, Poland
sorysz@student.agh.edu.pl

[2] II Department of Cardiology, Jakubowskiego 2, 30-688 Kraków, Poland

Abstract. First-generation contrast agents are used in echocardiography to diagnose PFO (Patent Foramen Ovale). The degree of PFO is based on the number of bubbles found in the left atrium. This paper presents research on the preparation of an algorithm for the segmentation of first-generation contrast bubbles. To fulfill the research objective, the images were first preprocessed to reduce the influence of possible noise and artefacts; subsequently, binarization was performed and the segmentation of bubbles then occurred. The results were evaluated by the Dice coefficient. To obtain the best results, the following local thresholding methods were compared: Median, Sauvola, and SDA. The outcome was evaluated and the best values of the Dice coefficient were obtained with two local thresholding methods: the Median and the Sauvola algorithms.

Keywords: Segmentation · Heart · Echocardiographic · PFO · Contrast

1 Introduction

Patent Foramen Ovale (PFO) is a relic of the foramen ovale, which exists between the left and right atria of the human fetus [1]. The foramen ovale is a hole during the fetal stage in the wall between the heart's atriums that is necessary for proper blood oxygenation [11]. In the two months after the birth of a child, it closes and thus forms the fossa ovalis [9,11]. However, in 20–25% of the population the overgrowth is not complete and the "cover" that closes the foramen ovale does not connect on one side of the hole, thereby creating a pathological connection whose degree of closure depends on the pressure in both atriums [9]. In most cases, there are no problems for patients with PFO in their day-to-day life [1]; however, complications arise if blood clots form, in which case there is a great risk of a vein obstruction in the brain that could lead to a stroke [1]. To prevent such incidents, diagnosis and prevention are required, and treatment is sometimes also needed. The aim of the initial examination is to determine the degree of PFO and the risk of occurrence of an obstruction. During this step, a transesophageal

N. Piaseczna et al. (Eds.): EMBS ICS 2020, AISC 1360, pp. 127–135, 2022.
https://doi.org/10.1007/978-3-030-88976-0_17

echocardiographic examination is performed with the use of a first-generation contrast agent; the assessment is based on the number of contrast bubbles in the left atrium [1]. Nowadays, this method is only performed manually by doctors; however, an automatic segmentation algorithm would allow the examination to be performed faster and with less effort. There have been no previous attempts to develop such a method, therefore this article aims to fill this gap. The results of the performed research are presented in this paper. The images were first preprocessed to reduce the influence of possible noise and artefacts; then binarization was performed, and finally the segmentation of bubbles occurred. The results were evaluated with the Dice coefficient [2]. To obtain the best results, local thresholding methods were compared: Median, Sauvola and SDA [3–7,10].

2 Materials and Methods

2.1 The Data

The datasets used in this research were provided by cardiologist Danuta Sorysz, MD, PhD; these were echocardiographic B-mode images acquired from different devices. Types of images collected were: grey-scale 16-bit, grey-scale 8-bit and RGB images (with grey-scale US image and color data about heart rate, etc.). The sets contained 4 images from 2 examinations which showed the heart from different angles and in different planes. In all of them, the left atrium and the wall between it and the right atrium were visible.

2.2 Methods

All the presented methods are implemented in ImageJ [8], which was used for the processing of the images.

Local Thresholding. Is a method that performs thresholding not on a whole image but on a neighborhood whose radius is indicated by the user. The algorithm that is used during the transformation is also chosen by the user. Auto Local Threshold is a set of methods in ImageJ, and the presented algorithms are unique to this platform. An important change that the authors of this plug-in made is that the neighborhoods are not rectangular (as in most original algorithms) but circular, therefore a radius is used instead of the length of the edges. The presented methods are part of the Local Thresholding group of functions.

Median. The threshold was calculated by subtracting the parameter C from the median value of each neighborhood. Then, each pixel's value in that neighborhood was compared with the threshold and assigned to one of two categories: object or background [4].

The Sauvola. Method is a variation of the Niblack algorithm that defines the threshold in a more efficient way. This method was created for thresholding mixed pages of text and images [7].

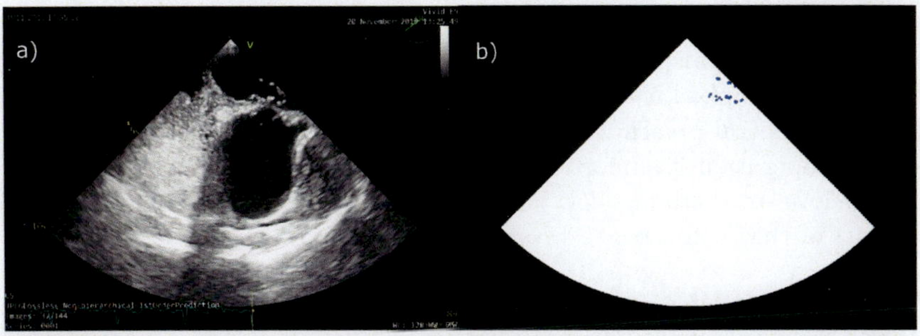

(a) a) Image A b) ROI with ground-truth for Image A

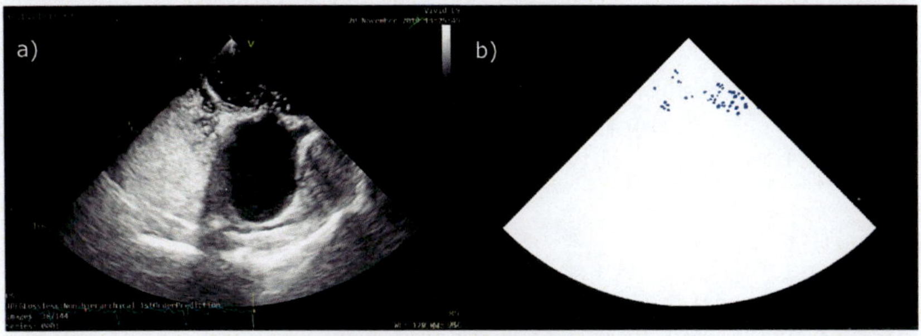

(b) a) Image B b) ROI with ground-truth for Image B

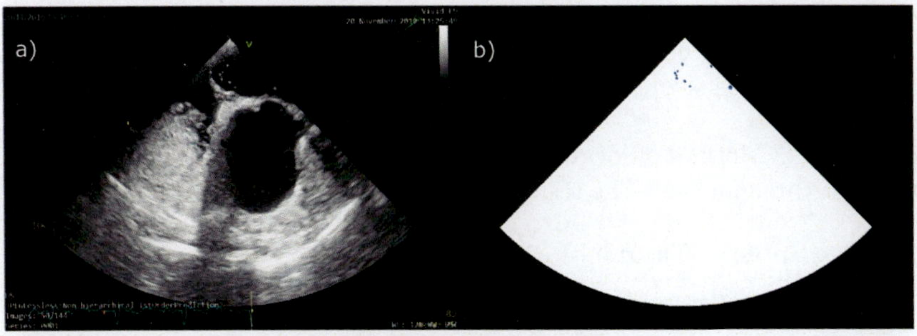

(c) a) Image C b) ROI with ground-truth for Image C

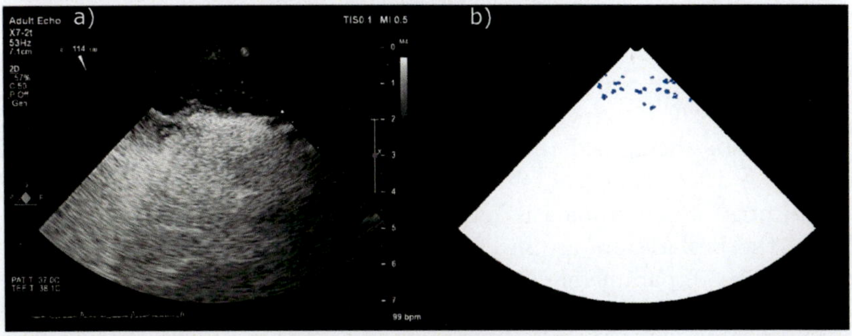

(d) a) Image D b) ROI with ground-truth for Image D

Fig. 1. Original images and corresponding manual segmentation (blue) and ROI (white)

Statistical Dominance Algorithm. (SDA) first counts the number of neighborhoods of a central pixel in the neighborhood of a user-defined radius. The final value of this pixel is the number of pixels whose values are greater than or equal to the central pixel's value. The output image is the result of a statistical dominance operation, therefore its values are correlated with the distribution of each grey level in the image [5]. Unlike the previous methods, this algorithm is not a part of the Auto Local Threshold function in ImageJ.

Dice Coefficient. Was used to evaluate the results of the experiment [10]. The algorithm for this process was based on this equation:

$$DSC = \frac{2TP}{2TP + FP + FN} \tag{1}$$

It was done by checking pixel-by-pixel values of the ground-truth image and the segmented one, where TP is true positive, FP is false positive, FN is false negative and FP is false positive.

3 Results

The four original images (Fig. 1) were processed with the use of the aforementioned methods. After the SDA algorithm, the final binarization step was performed; the other two methods performed thresholding during their processing. The results are presented as follows: first, the graphs and results for each method and image; second, a comparison table for each image; lastly, the best methods, parameters and the segmented images.

The Median. Method of local thresholding gave the best Dice coefficient values for the first three images. The results for all four images are presented in Table 1.

Table 1. The results of the Median method for all images

Image	Parameters	Dice coefficient
A	Radius 7, parameter C-88	0.646
B	Radius 7, parameter C-54	0.5749
C	Radius 7, parameter C-88	0.646
D	Radius 8, parameter C-58	0.2521

It should be mentioned that for image D, most of the methods produced relatively low Dice coefficient values; therefore, it should not be surprising that the result presented in Table 1 is lower than for all other images. As can be seen in Fig. 2, the best results are inversely proportional to the radius and are for negative values of parameter C.

Sauvola. Is the other algorithm that produced a very good outcome; its results are presented in Table 2. A graphical representation of the results is presented in Fig. 3. The grate surprise presents the result for image D, as it is greater then 0.6.

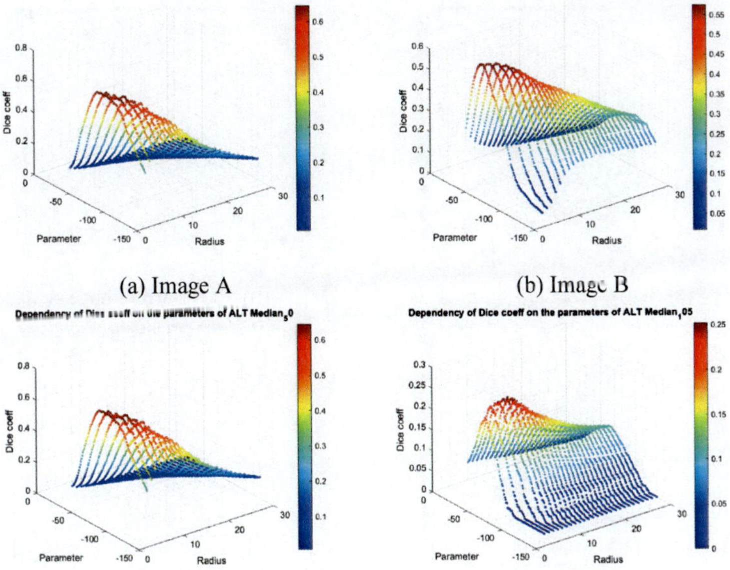

(a) Image A (b) Image B

(c) Image C (d) Image D

Fig. 2. Graphic representation of searched planes of the parameters for Median method

Table 2. The results of the Sauvola method for all images

Image	Parameters	Dice coefficient
A	Radius 13, KV-2.35 RV 0	0.3684
B	Radius 15, KV-2.35 RV 0	0.4016
C	Radius 12, KV-3 RV 0	0.4119
D	Radius 25, KV-0.1 RV-0.8	0.6278

SDA. The last method also produced good results. Table 3 and Fig. 4 show the results of processing all images with the SDA method. The best result was obtained for the image C with the disc neighborhood and parameters: SDA threshold 45 and radius 13.

Table 3. The best results of the SDA method for each image

Image	Neighborhood	Parameters	Dice coefficient
A	Disc	SDAt 75 radius 12	0.5747
B	Snowflake	SDAt 141 radius 50	0.5537
C	Disc	SDAt 45 radius 13	0.6810
D	Disc	SDAt 34 radius 13	0.4074

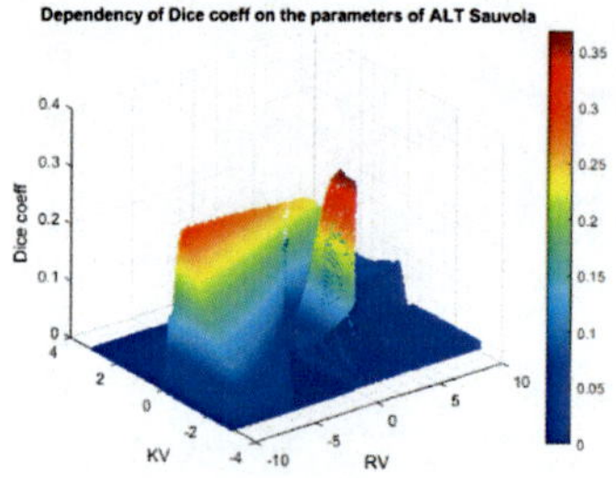

(a) Sauvola(KV, RV) Image A

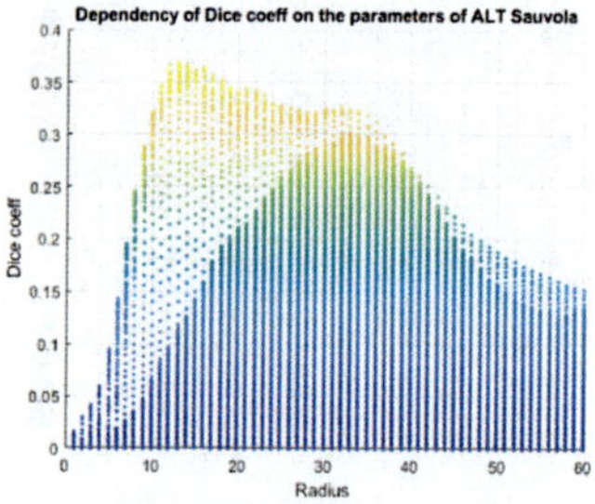

(b) Sauvola(R) Image A

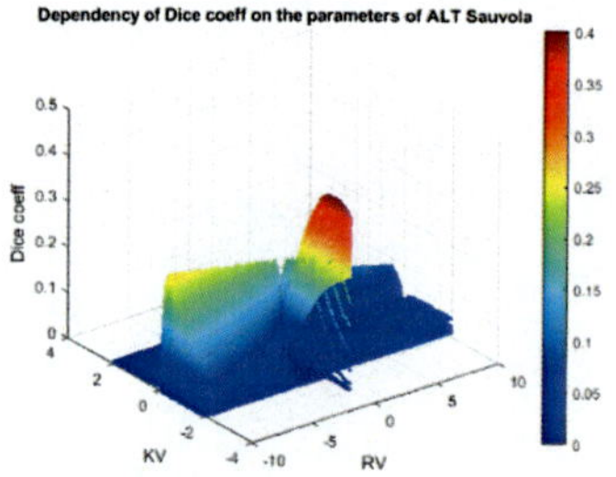

(c) Sauvola(KV, RV) Image B

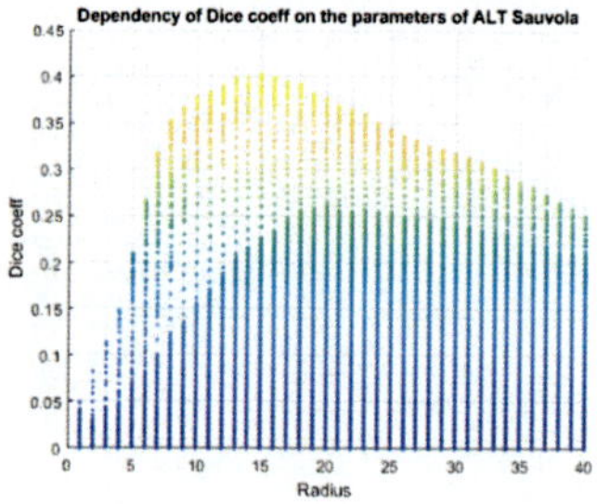

(d) Sauvola(R) Image B

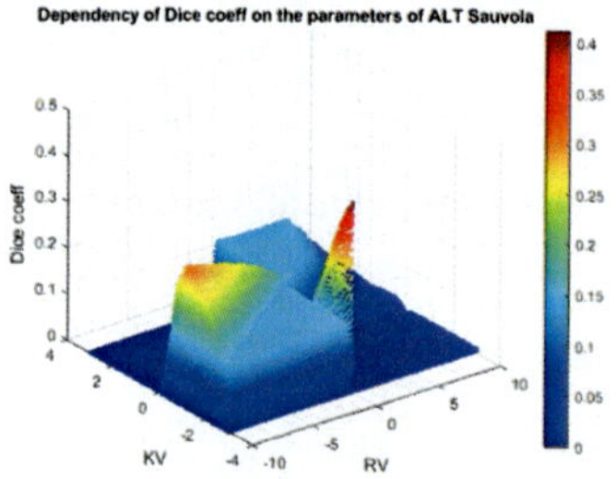

(e) Sauvola(KV, RV) Image C

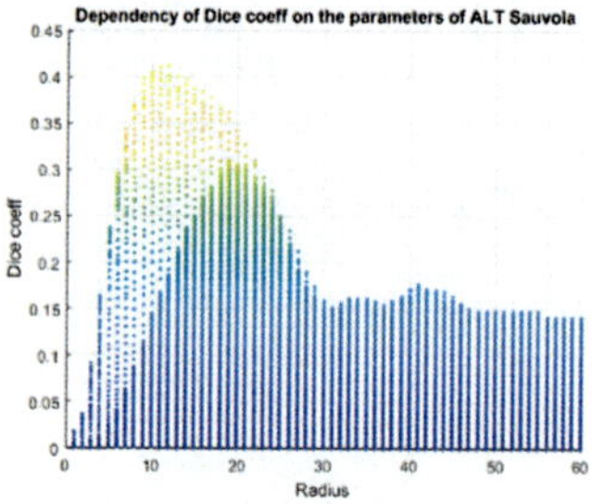

(f) Sauvola(R) Image C

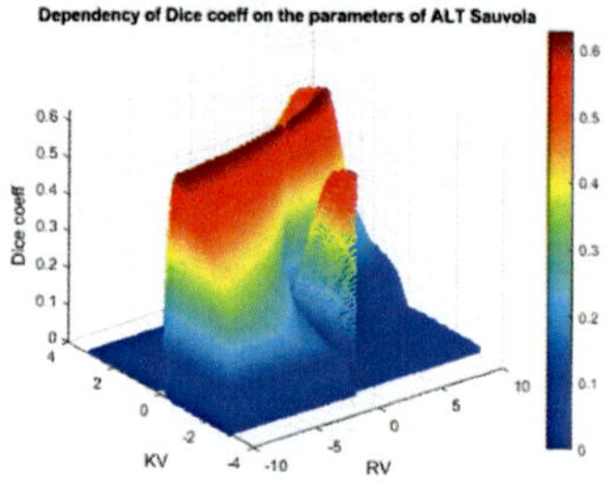

(g) Sauvola(KV, RV) Image D

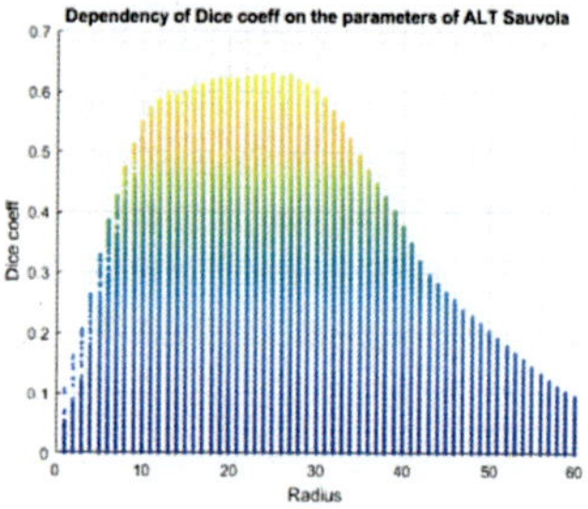

(h) Sauvola(R) Image D

Fig. 3. Graphic representation of the searched planes of the parameters for the Sauvola method. a), c) and e) present the dependency on the RV and KV parameters; b), d) and f) present the dependency on the radius

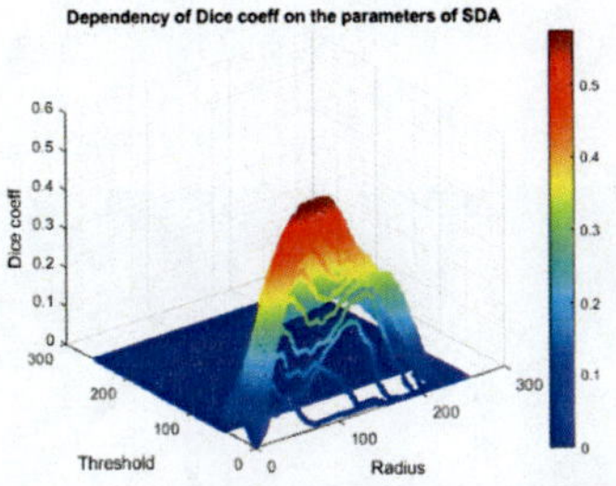

(a) SDA(R, Thr) disc Image A

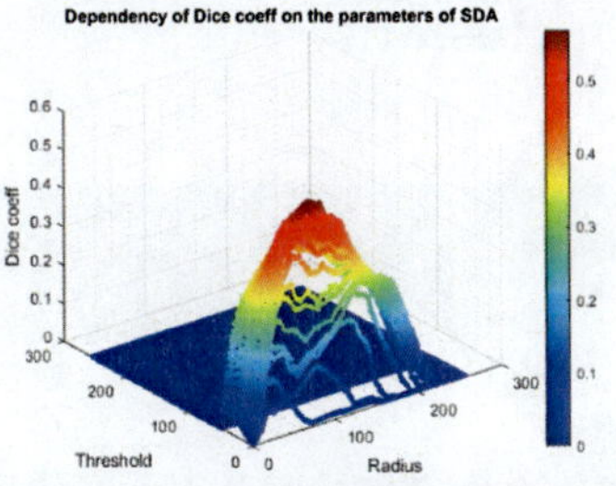

(b) SDA(R, Thr) snow Image A

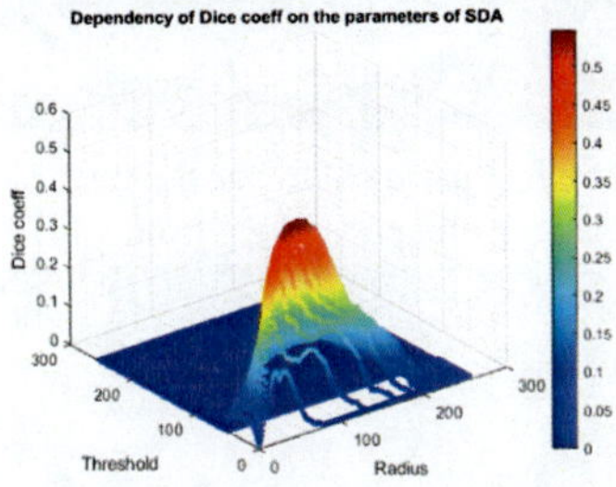

(c) SDA(R, Thr) disc Image B

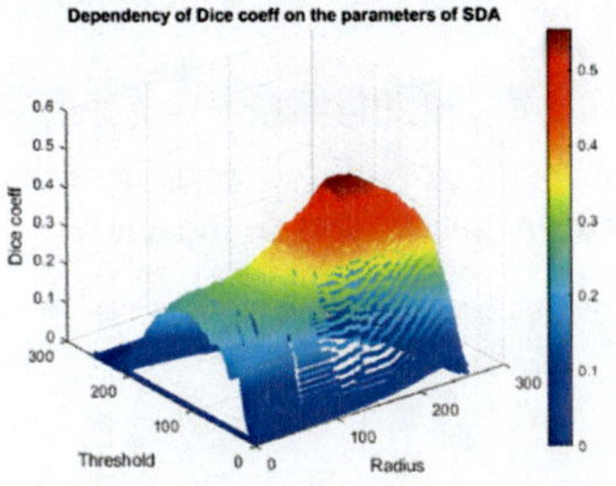

(d) SDA(R, Thr) snow Image B

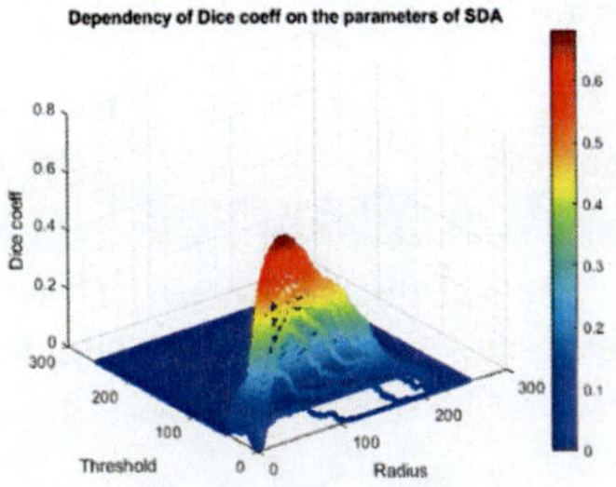

(e) SDA(R, Thr) disc Image C

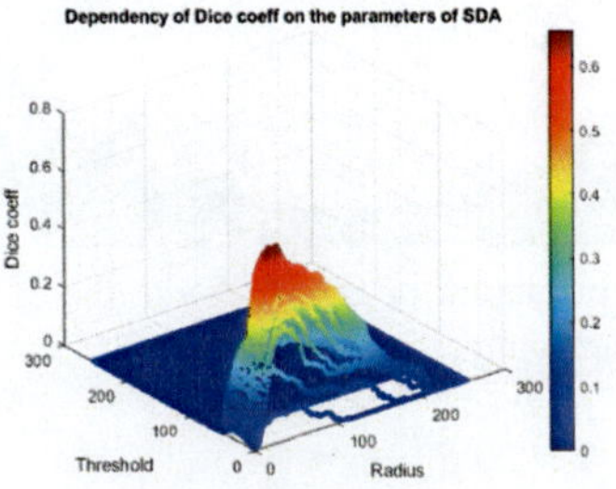

(f) SDA(R, Thr) snow Image C

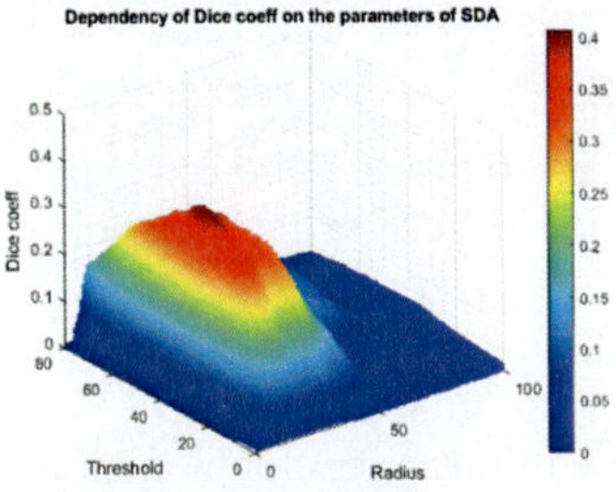

(g) SDA(R, Thr) disc Image D

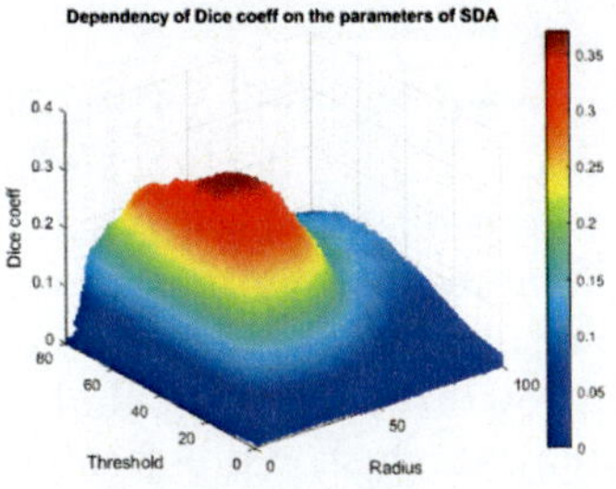

(h) SDA(R, Thr) snow Image D

Fig. 4. Graphic representation of the results of the SDA method. a), c) e) and g) presents the dependency on the SDA threshold and radius for disc neighborhood; b), d), f) and h) presents the dependency on the SDA threshold and radius for snowflake neighborhood

4 Conclusions

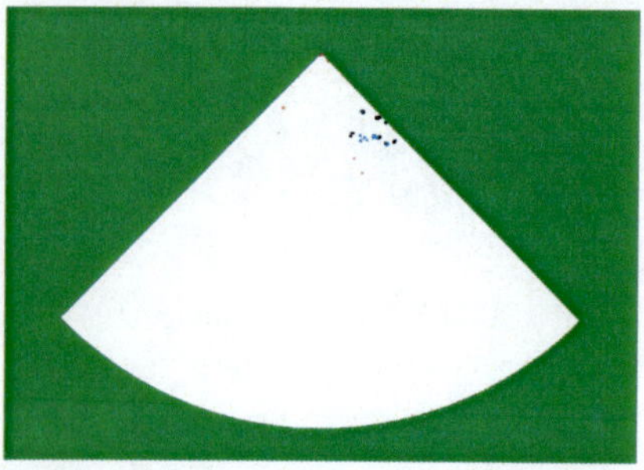

(a) Segmentation of Image A with the Median algorithm and parameters from table 1

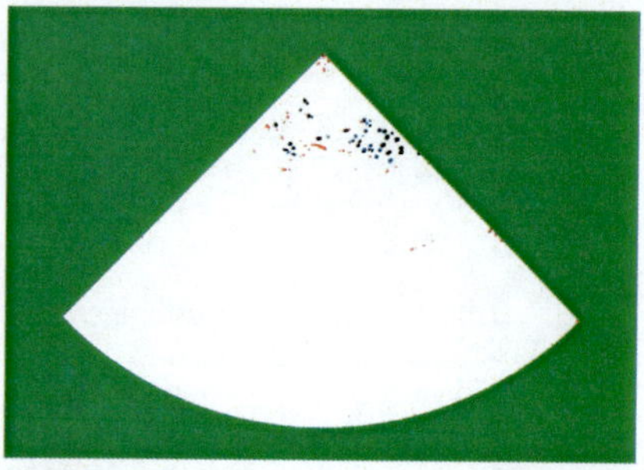

(b) Segmentation of Image B with the Median algorithm and parameters from table 1

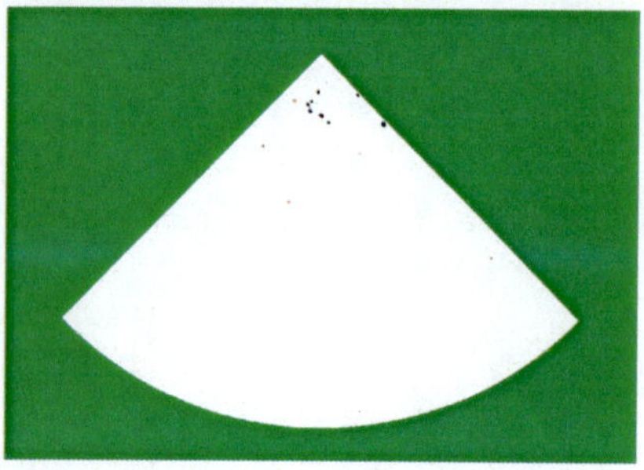

(c) Segmentation of Image C with the SDA algorithm and parameters from table 3

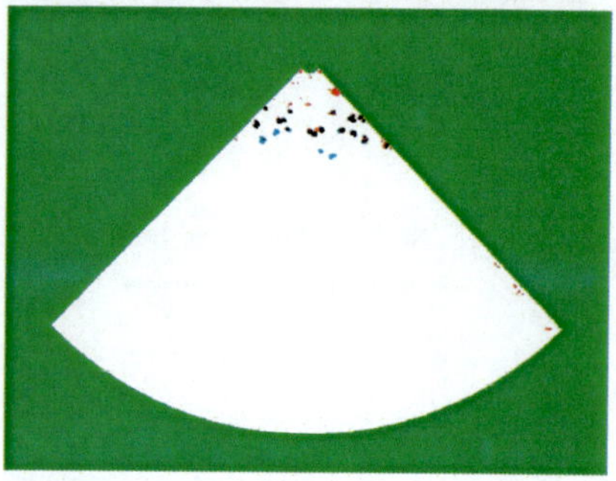

(d) Segmentation of Image D with the Sauvola algorithm and parameters from table 2

Fig. 5. The best segmentations for each image

Figure 5 presents the original segmented images. The processing method used was the one that gave the best result for a given image. The coloring scheme is as follows: green is the background, light blue is false negative results, black is true positive results, red indicates false positive results, and white shows true negative results. As can be easily seen in these images, the selected algorithms produced good results that could be used in the final algorithm.

Future research should be conducted to check the results of combined local-thresholding methods such as Median, Sauvola, and SDA, as these look very promising.

Acknowledgements. This publication was funded by AGH University of Science and Technology, Faculty of Electrical Engineering, Automatics, Computer Science and Biomedical Engineering.

References

1. Bang, O.Y., Lee, M.J., Ryoo, S., Kim, S.J., Kim, J.W.: Patent foramen ovale and stroke-current status. J. stroke **17**(3), 229 (2015)
2. Dice, L.R.: Measures of the amount of ecologic association between species. Ecology **26**(3), 297–302 (1945)
3. Nichele, L., Persichetti, V., Lucidi, M., Cincotti, G.: Quantitative evaluation of ImageJ thresholding algorithms for microbial cell counting. OSA Continuum **3**(6), 1417–1427 (2020). https://doi.org/10.1364/OSAC.393971
4. Otsu, N.: A threshold selection method from gray-scale histogram. IEEE Trans. Syst., Man, Cyber **1**, 62–66 (1998)
5. Piórkowski, A.: A statistical dominance algorithm for edge detection and segmentation of medical images. In: Piętka, E., Badura, P., Kawa, J., Wieclawek, W. (eds.) Information Technologies in Medicine. AISC, vol. 471, pp. 3–14. Springer, Cham (2016). https://doi.org/10.1007/978-3-319-39796-2_1
6. Sage, D., Unser, M.: Easy java programming for teaching image-processing. In: Proceedings 2001 International Conference on Image Processing, vol. 3, pp. 298–301. IEEE (2001)
7. Sauvola, J., Pietikäinen, M.: Adaptive document image binarization. Pattern Recogn. **33**(2), 225–236 (2000)
8. Schneider, C.A., Rasband, W.S., Eliceiri, K.W.: NIH Image to ImageJ: 25 years of image analysis. Nat. Methods **9**(7), 671–675 (2012)
9. Silvestry, F.E., et al.: Guidelines for the echocardiographic assessment of atrial septal defect and patent foramen ovale: from the american society of echocardiography and society for cardiac angiography and interventions. J. Am. Soc. Echocardiogr. **28**(8), 910–958 (2015)
10. Sorensen, T.A.: A method of establishing groups of equal amplitude in plant sociology based on similarity of species content and its application to analyses of the vegetation on danish commons. Biol. Skar. **5**, 1–34 (1948)
11. Yee, K., Lui, F.: Anatomy, Thorax, Heart Foramen Ovale. StatPearls, pMID: 31424787 (2020)

Check for updates

Measurement of CO_2 Retention in Subea EasyBreath Masks Converted into Improvised COVID19 Protection Measures for Medical Services

Juliusz Stefański[1(✉)], Olaf Tomaszewski[1], Marek Iwaniec[2], and Jacek Wesół[2]

[1] "BioMetr" Student Science Club, AGH University of Science and Technology, Cracow, Poland
juliusz@stefanscy.pl

[2] Department of Process Control, Faculty of Mechanical Engineering and Robotics, AGH University of Science and Technology, Cracow, Poland

Abstract. Studies of 9 volunteers wearing a full-face mask were carried out to measure changes in CO_2 concentration, pressure, air volume, and temperature. Each volunteer had a total of 6 measurements taken either while sitting or performing physical activity (walking at a speed of 4.5 km/h). The masks were converted from the SNORKELING EASYBREATH 500 SUBEA model purchased in the DECATHLON chain of stores, they were given to paramedics, and a few were left for testing. The proposed solution includes an application that acquires, processes, visualizes, and stores the signals understudy, and an electronic system to collect the parameters described above. Python was used to create the program due to its extensive number of signal analysis libraries. The measuring system is based on the ESP32 devkit V1 microcontroller. It is a popular choice for prototyping measuring systems. As part of our campaign called "Przyłbica dla Medyka AGH" (face shield for medic AGH), tests have been carried out since May, in cooperation with medical centers throughout the country. About 10,000 full face masks have already been handed over to healthcare professionals. We hope that the solutions we propose using the Internet of Things (IoT) technology will increase the comfort of the work of medical personnel throughout the country.

Keywords: Protection measures · Carbon dioxide · Measuring system · COVID19

1 Introduction

Carbon dioxide (CO_2) is a colorless, odorless, and non-flammable gas at room temperature. Paramedics should pay special attention to the prevention of CO_2 poisoning at the time of a rescue operation if such a risk occurs. Increased and prolonged exposure to carbon dioxide at elevated concentrations may result in

N. Piaseczna et al. (Eds.): EMBS ICS 2020, AISC 1360, pp. 136–143, 2022.
https://doi.org/10.1007/978-3-030-88976-0_18

the necessity of evacuating a paramedic as soon as possible to the area where the air composition is safer. Overdosing CO_2 in breathable air may result in symptoms such as: a sharp decline in cognitive abilities, respiratory failure, and cardiac arrest. Although carbon dioxide poisoning is relatively rare, it is good practice to have it verified in an emergency room [1].

The assumed carbon dioxide content in the (outside) inhaled air is 410 ppm (0.041%), while in the exhaled air it is approximately 40000 ppm (4%). Regarding ventilated rooms, these values fluctuate (depending on the current number of people) around 5000–20000 ppm (0.5–2%) of CO_2. According to The National Institute for Occupational Safety and Health, a 30-min exposure at 50,000 ppm produces signs of intoxication and a few minutes of exposure at 70,000 ppm and 100,000 ppm produces unconsciousness (Fig. 1).

2 Materials and Methods

Due to the OHS concerns, one volunteer was tested daily in a mask with a measuring system. Together with mask adapters, special valves were designed in cooperation with Maska dla Medyka [2] design team to reduce CO_2 levels in the intake air. We start the test with the valve attached while sitting for 5–10 min, then 10 min without the valve attached. Then, the treadmill exercise test (Fig. 3) is performed at a speed of 4.5 km/h. The examined person exercised for 5–10 min in a mask with a valve and 10 min in a mask without a valve. Finally, the volunteer sits down on a chair and a reference measurement is taken in a commercial half-mask for 10 min and without a mask for 5 min. During the experiment, there are rest and hydration breaks of up to 3 min between measurements. After all, the mask, half-mask, and tube are disinfected with special care in a gutter with a disinfectant liquid.

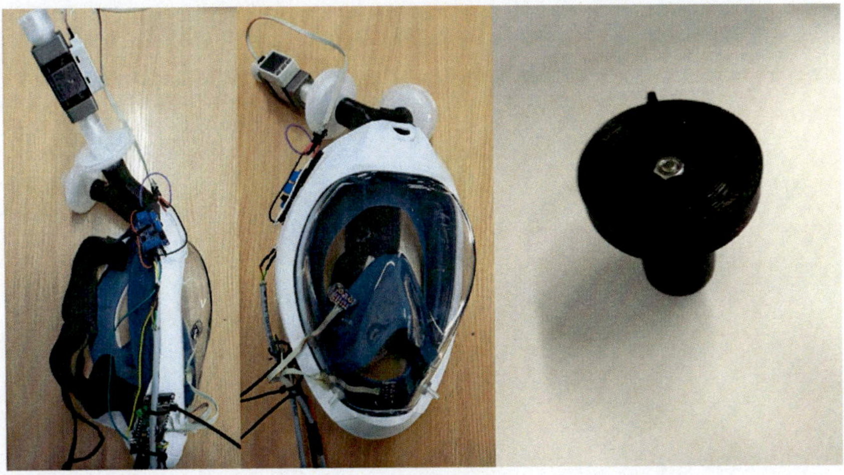

Fig. 1. Mask used during the trials and 3D printed valve used in measurements.

The full-face mask used has the following dimensions: height: 28 cm, width: 18 cm, thickness: 12 cm. The mask weighs 600 g. During the tests, the volume of inhaled air, changes in CO_2 concentration, changes in pressure, and temperature are examined. According to the documentation on the manufacturer's website, there may be problems with the tightness of the mask when the test person has facial hair [3] (Fig. 2).

The measuring system consists of the ESP32 Devkit v1 [4] microcontroller to which are connected CO_2 sensors [5], temperature-pressure [6], and a flow meter [7]. The data is downloaded with a frequency 20 Hz and sent via the USB port to the computer. Since the signal from the flowmeter is 4–20 mA standard,

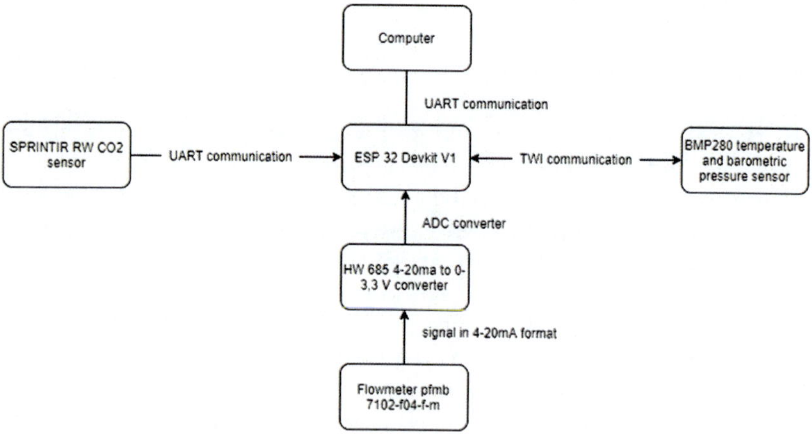

Fig. 2. Scheme of the measurement system.

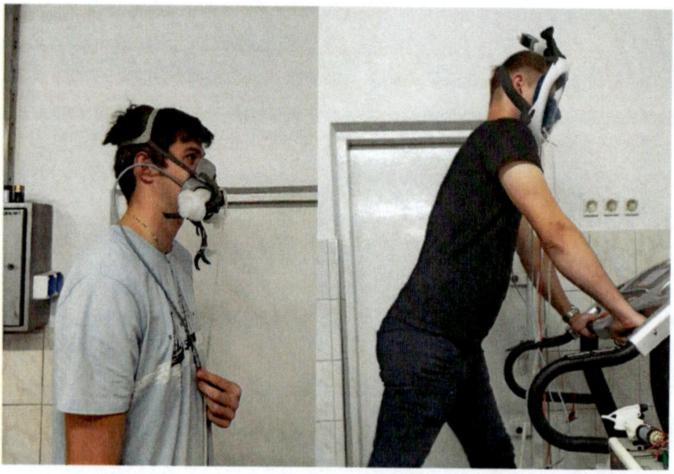

Fig. 3. Volunteers wearing a commercial half mask and modified SUBEA mask with the valve attached during measurements.

we decided to use a 4–20 mA to a 0–3.3 Vm converter which we read using an analog-to-digital converter built into the microcontroller.

For this paper, 9 volunteers were successfully tested and the results of their measurements were included in this paper.

3 Results

The raw signal was filtered with a 10th order Butterworth low pass filter with a cut-off frequency of 5 Hz. Then the Hilbert transform was used to calculate its envelope. The local maxima and minima of the envelope were used to calculate the mean, maximum, and minimum saturation of CO_2 inside the mask. It was then used to compare masks with 3D printed valves, to masks without them, and to reference values. Figure 4 shows the 160 s window of raw signal with envelope and inspiratory curves fitted to a minimum and maximum values of CO_2 for volunteer 2 walking with a mask fitted with 3D printed valve (Fig. 5, 6).

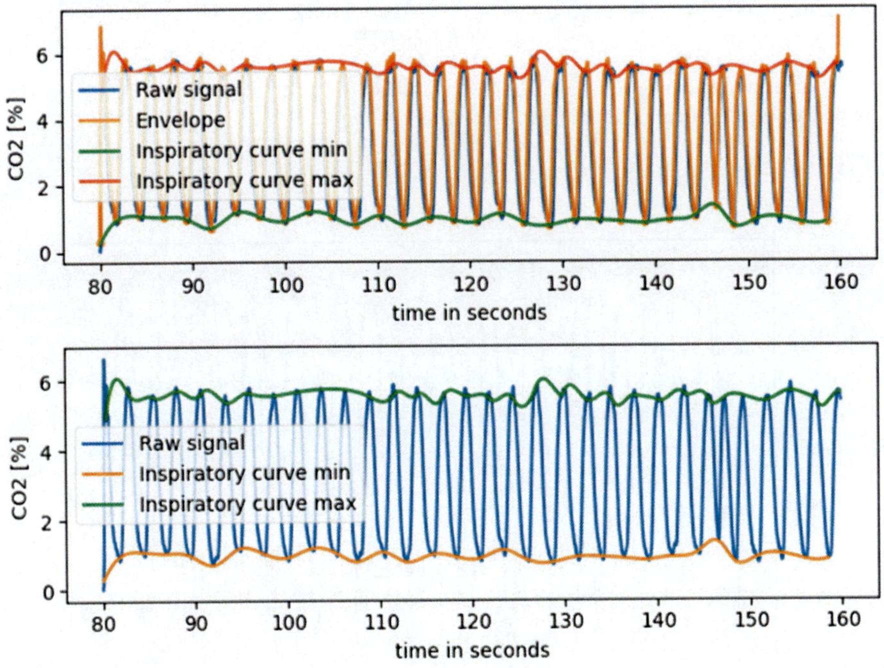

Fig. 4. Graph of the signal acquired from the CO_2 sensor for the measurement of the filter mask with envelope, and inspiratory curves fitted to a minimum and maximum values of CO_2 for volunteer 2 walking with a mask fitted with 3D printed valve.

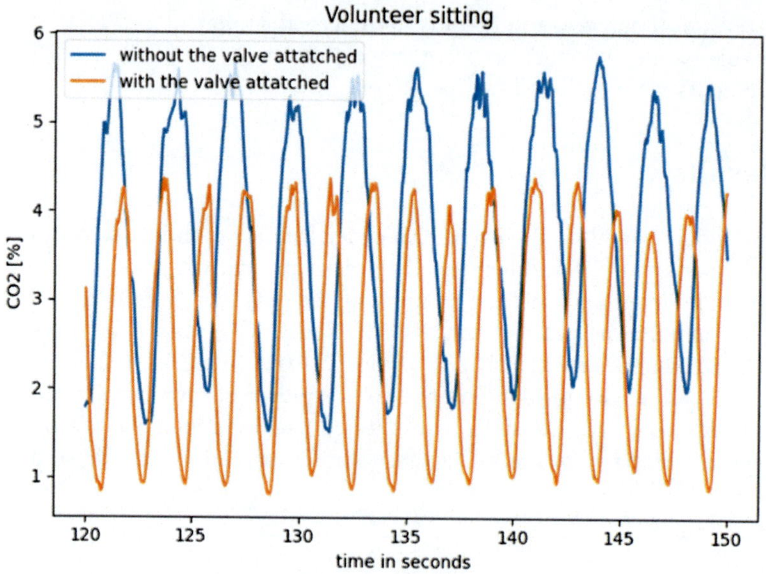

Fig. 5. Graph of the fragment of the signal acquired from the volunteer 2 sitting wearing a mask with and without attached 3D printed valve.

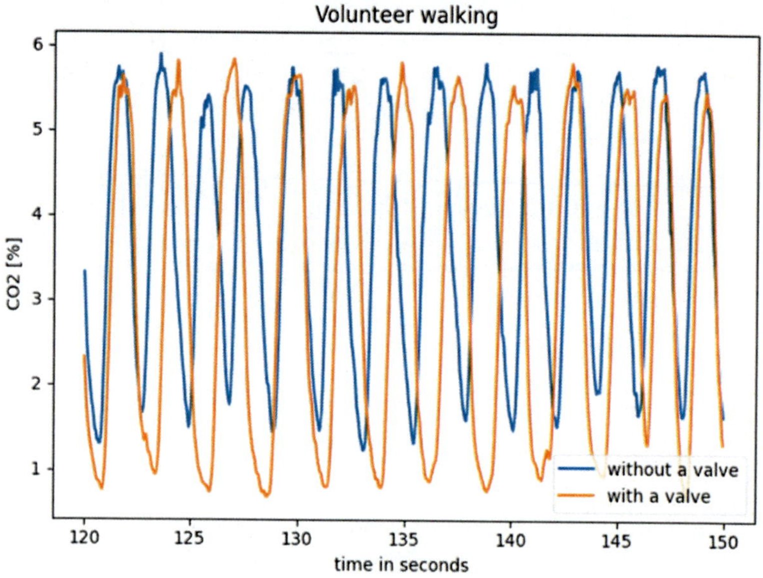

Fig. 6. Graph of the fragment of the signal acquired from the volunteer 2 walking wearing a mask with and without attached 3D printed valve.

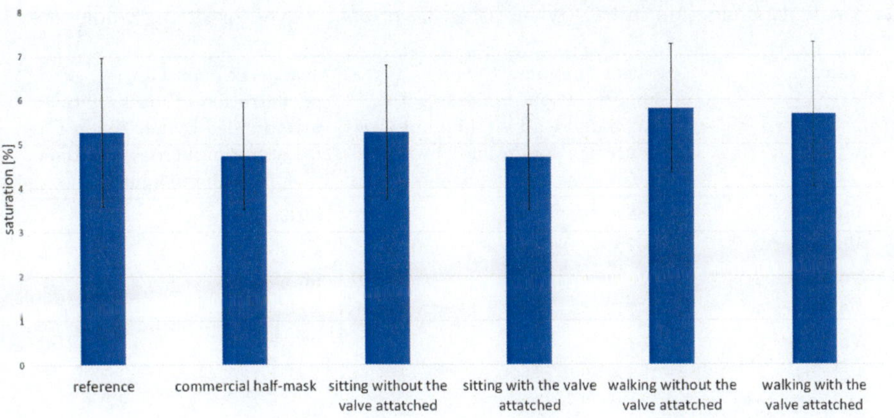

Fig. 7. Mean values with standard deviation acquired for maximum CO_2 levels for all 9 volunteers.

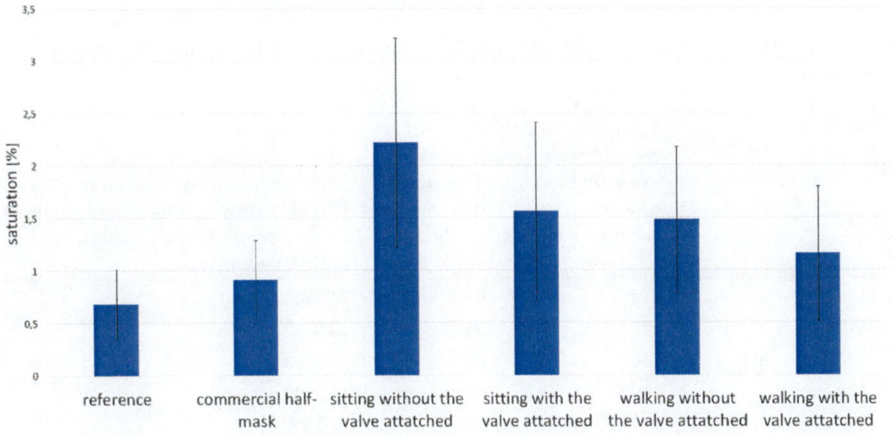

Fig. 8. Mean values with standard deviation acquired for minimum CO_2 levels for all 9 volunteers.

Table 1. Reduction in CO_2 when using 3D printed valves for sitting volunteers.

Value	Mean minimum CO_2 concentration in masks with valve divided by minimum CO_2 concentration in masks without valve in sitting volunteers	Mean maximum CO_2 concentration in masks with valve divided by maximum CO_2 concentration in masks without valve in sitting volunteers
Volunteer 1	88%	89%
Volunteer 2	47%	81%
Volunteer 3	55%	96%
Volunteer 4	67%	82%
Volunteer 5	61%	93%
Volunteer 6	109%	110%
Volunteer 7	88%	83%
Volunteer 8	62%	91%
Volunteer 9	60%	137%
Mean values	70%	96%
Standard deviation	20%	18%

Table 2. Reduction in CO_2 when using 3D printed valves for volunteers walking on the treadmill.

Value	Mean minimum CO_2 concentration in masks with valve divided by minimum CO_2 concentration in masks without valve in volunteers walking on the treadmill	Mean maximum CO_2 concentration in masks with valve divided by maximum CO_2 concentration in masks without valve in volunteers walking on the treadmill
Volunteer 1	74%	99%
Volunteer 2	51%	102%
Volunteer 3	85%	101%
Volunteer 4	80%	98%
Volunteer 5	117%	94%
Volunteer 6	83%	90%
Volunteer 7	93%	102%
Volunteer 8	53%	88%
Volunteer 9	63%	92%
Mean values	78%	96%
Standard deviation	21%	5%

4 Conclusion

The presence of valves correlates with CO_2 level reduction. Due to a high standard deviation in the results (Figs. 7 and 8), the team calculated CO_2 difference for each volunteer when using a mask with a 3D printed valve. Tables 1 and 2 show the difference. The exercise of treadmill walking is accompanied by an increase in breathing frequency and lung ventilation. As lung ventilation increases, the effect of valves on the minimum CO_2 concentration decreases. It is assumed that the valves affect the respiratory rate and the volume of air inhaled. Subsequent studies will examine these parameters.

The biggest flaw of the used masks is their size. Because there is only a single model available, some volunteers with smaller faces were unable to obtain a sealed fit, resulting in a measurable backdraft of exhaust air. Therefore, both the orinasal and facial parts of the mask were acting as a dead space. The same issue was encountered for males with facial hair.

In 2020, due to their low cost and accessibility, over 10 000 of SNORKELING EASYBREATH 500 SUBEA masks were converted in Poland to be used by medical personnel [8]. The above results confirmed, that the values of CO_2 are in an acceptable range and that 3D printed valves help with reduction of the CO_2 levels in inhaled air. While the masks can't be used by everyone in the time of pandemic they were available in high quantity and the process of modification was fairly inexpensive.

References

1. The National Institute for Occupational Safety and Health (NIOSH). https://www.cdc.gov/niosh/idlh/124389.html. Accessed 10 Jan 2020
2. Maska dla Medyka (mask for medic) website. https://www.maskadlamedyka.pl/. Accessed 10 Jan 2020
3. Decathlon store. https://www.decathlon.pl/p/maska-powierzchniowa-do-snorkelingu-easybreath-500-oyster/_/R-p-148873. Accessed 10 Jan 2020
4. ESP32 documentation. https://www.espressif.com/sites/default/files/documentation/esp32_datasheet_en.pdf. Accessed 10 Jan 2020
5. CO_2 sensor documentation. https://www.gassensing.co.uk/wp-content/uploads/2020/07/SprintIR-W-Data-Sheet-Rev-4.3.pdf. Accessed 10 Jan 2020
6. BMP280 datasheet. http://domoticx.com/wp-content/uploads/2018/04/BMP280-datasheet-bosch.pdf. Accessed 10 Jan 2020
7. Flowmeter documentation. https://content2.smcetech.com/pdf/Manuals/PF-OMP0002-G.pdf. Accessed 10 Jan 2020
8. Maska dla Medyka, over 10 000 masks bought to support medical facilities in Poland. https://centrumdruku3d.pl/maskadlamedyka-10-tys-masek-dla-sluzby-zdrowia-dzieki-wsparciu-wosp-i-polskich-firm/. Accessed 10 Jan 2020

Selection of Interpretable *Decision Tree* as a Method for Classification of Early and Developed Glaucoma

Dominika Sułot(✉)

Department of Biomedical Engineering, Wroclaw University of Science and Technology, Wybrzeże Stanisława Wyspiańskiego 27, 50-370 Wrocław, Poland
dominika.sulot@pwr.edu.pl

Abstract. The purpose is to develop a pattern recognition model that would be able to classify three groups of glaucoma progression (which are: healthy controls, glaucoma suspects, and glaucoma patients) while being interpretable by medical doctors, being non-expert in machine learning. The utilized dataset is a numerical collection of 48 biomarkers acquired from each of 211 patients classified into three groups by an ophthalmologist. Due to the numerical type of the features and the high need for interpretability, it was decided to employ *Classification and Regression Trees*, and optimize them to obtain the smallest possible number of nodes and thus the highest interpretability while maintaining statistical dependence to the model with the highest quality metric from the review. The 5×5 cross-validation protocol was used in the designed and conducted experiments. Two criteria were validated to assess the quality of the model selection – *balanced accuracy* metric and the number of nodes in the tree. The results indicate that this fairly simple approach could preserve a high *balanced accuracy* score and simultaneously reduce the size of the model – thereby increasing its interpretability. For $\alpha = 0.2$, this approach can reduce the size of the *Classification and Regression Trees* to a quarter of its original spread.

Keywords: Glaucoma classification · Classification and regression trees · Model interpretability

1 Introduction

Early detection of glaucoma is increasingly important as it is ranked as the second leading cause of blindness in the world. Glaucoma is a group of eye diseases and the main division into its types is based on the drainage angle. A distinction is made between *open-angle* and *angle-closure* glaucoma. While *angle-closure* glaucoma causes a sudden increase in intraocular pressure (IOP), *open-angle* glaucoma, which is the most common type, develops slowly and asymptomatically over the years, therefore it is usually detected at a stage where its effects cannot

N. Piaseczna et al. (Eds.): EMBS ICS 2020, AISC 1360, pp. 144–150, 2022.
https://doi.org/10.1007/978-3-030-88976-0_19

be undone [1,2], making it a diagnostic challenge. This type is being considered in this paper and will be referred to as glaucoma. To prevent irreversible damage to the optic nerve, methods for early glaucoma detection are needed. For this purpose, the group of so-called glaucoma suspects is most often used. It includes patients who are not yet clinically symptomatic but have a glaucomatous optic disk appearance while having not elevated IOP. This type will in most cases lead to the development of glaucoma in the future, so detecting it and attempting to control the disease is essential [3].

Along with the development of new technologies and algorithms, machine learning is increasingly used to support medical diagnostics. In the diagnosis of glaucoma, it is especially useful for determining the retinal nerve fiber layer (RNFL) thickness and other biomarkers from images obtained with optical coherence tomography (OCT) [4–6]. It is also increasingly often used to support decisions about the occurrence of a given disease [7,8]. Although many advanced techniques, some based on deep learning, for supporting glaucoma diagnosis have been continuously developed [8,9], the decision whether a patient has a glaucomatous eye is decided by a trained ophthalmologist based essentially on two critical parameters, i.e., the thickness of the retinal nerve fiber layer and the outcome of the visual filed [10]. However, in the case of machine learning solutions, usually for people who are not the authors of the solution or are not familiar with the technical basics of machine learning, it is simply a black box that classifies data without giving the basis of the decision. This is where the problem of interpretability arises. In the case of medical problems and health care, where ultimately medical doctors and medical staff are supposed to use these solutions, an important factor is to focus on the issue of the interpretability of the models and of the results obtained by them [11,12].

2 Methods

2.1 Dataset

In this paper, retrospective data collection is used [13]. It consists of numerical values of biomarkers that are usually acquired while evaluating glaucoma. A study in which data from subjects were collected, was approved by the Bioethical Committee of the Wroclaw Medical University (KB–332/2015) and adhered to the tenets of the Declaration of Helsinki. Informed written consent to participate was obtained from all subjects. For each subject, 48 features were obtained, on the basis of which, and on the basis of the eye image made with the use of OCT, an experienced ophthalmologist assigned them to one of the three groups. Among the features considered, the following can be distinguished: a) RNFL thickness, measured in six sectors, as well as the average value of those sectors, b) age of the patient, c) the value of intraocular pressure, d) field of view measurement result, e) lamina cribrosa depth and shape, and others. Full details of each of the features collected and the course of medical examination data can be found in [13].

The analyzed data were acquired from 211 patients. Each of the subjects was classified into one of the three groups. Finally, the distribution of the number in the given groups was as follows: 69 – healthy controls, 72 – glaucoma suspects, and 70 glaucoma patients.

Since the number of patients is small, and each of them has a large number of features, based on which the classification is to be performed, a phenomenon called *the curse of dimensionality* may occur. It consists in the fact that with the increase in the dimensionality of the data, the need for a larger number of learning patterns increases, which in this case cannot be met. This problem will be considered later in the paper.

2.2 Classification and Regression Trees

Considering the high need for interpretability and data in the form of numerical values, it was decided, in this paper, to use *Classification and Regression Trees* (CART) [14] for the classification task. It is an algorithm first introduced in 1984. The operating principle is based on the continuous partitioning of data according to the Gini impurity measure through a process known as *binary recursive partitioning.* The great advantage of this algorithm is also the ability to control its parameters at the learning stage, e.g., the depth of the created tree. This feature of the algorithm was used to differentiate the models.

3 Design of Experiment

The entire experiment was conducted using Python 3.8.6 language and the scikit-learn 0.23.2 library [15].

Due to the *curse of dimensionality*, it was decided to use preprocessing which reduced the number of features for each patient. For this purpose, the ANOVA test was utilized [16]. The F-values obtained for each feature are shown in Fig. 1. After preliminary analysis, it was noticed that many of the available features do not differentiate the classes like the others, so for further experiments, it was decided to select only the 20 most differentiable out of the 48 available features. With the usage of the rest of the data, the set of CART classifiers was trained using 5×5–fold repeated cross-validation protocol and the whole analysis was conducted using the average value of those folds. The simple grid search optimization protocol [17] was used to conduct a complete review of 20 quants for each of the three analyzed parameters of the tree, which are: a) a maximum depth of the tree, b) a minimum number of samples required to split an internal node, and c) a maximum number of features to consider when looking for the best split. For a and c, the values of the quants were linearly distributed in the range from 1 to 20. For b, the values were a linear distribution ranging from 1 to 99%.

The next step was the selection of the best tree from the complete review, that would meet both the requirements of interpretability and high accuracy. It was decided to use two criteria based on which the trees were assessed. The first one,

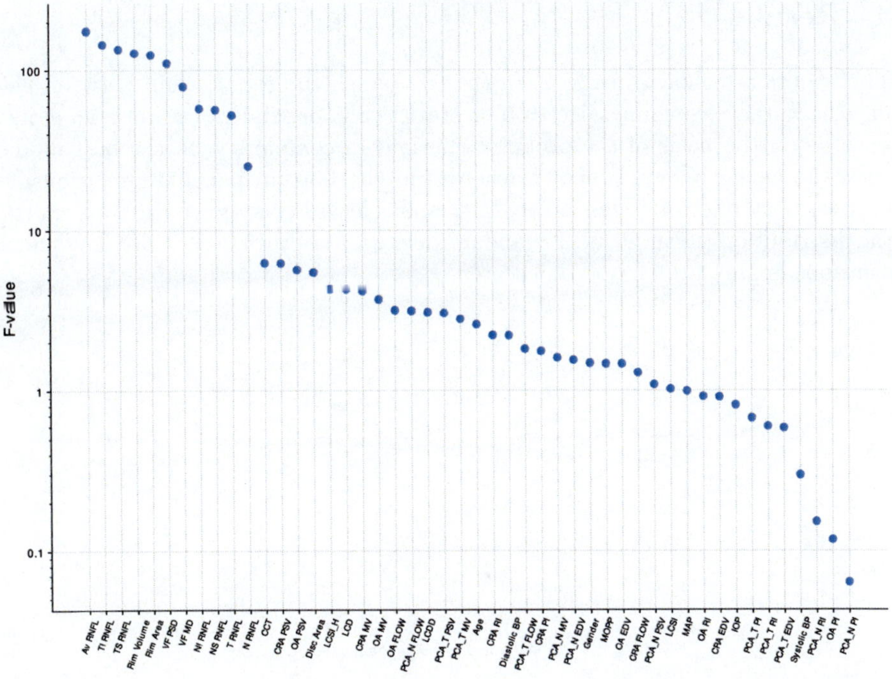

Fig. 1. The obtained F-values for individual features from the dataset using ANOVA on a logarithmic scale.

balanced accuracy score is calculated as the arithmetic mean of sensitivity and specificity and determines the accuracy of the trained model in the classification of new, unknown objects [18]. The second one, the number of nodes in the tree, determines how easily the tree will be interpreted because the smaller the tree the easier it is.

For each of the trained models, both of these criteria were calculated. The tree that achieved the best *balanced accuracy* (after averaging over the folds) was marked as *the best* tree in the review and the next steps of the experiment were referenced to it.

Having a complete review and the best model based on *balanced accuracy*, the set of statistically dependent models for the best one was selected based on *corrected t-test* [19]. For this purpose, a range of different *statistical significance level* (α) values were considered to see how this value would affect the final selection result. The final step of the proposed method was to select from this subset of dependent models that model that had the smallest number of nodes, i.e., the highest interpretability. This model is annotated as *optimally the best.*

4 Results

The results are shown in Fig. 2. In the top panel, the relationship between *balanced accuracy score* and selected α on statistically dependent results from model selected on the basis of the proposed method in comparison to the best model from the whole review is shown whereas in the bottom panel the relationship between a number of nodes in the CART and selected α is shown. In both charts, the distribution (mean value $\pm$ standard deviation) of the statistically dependent solutions is presented as a shaded area.

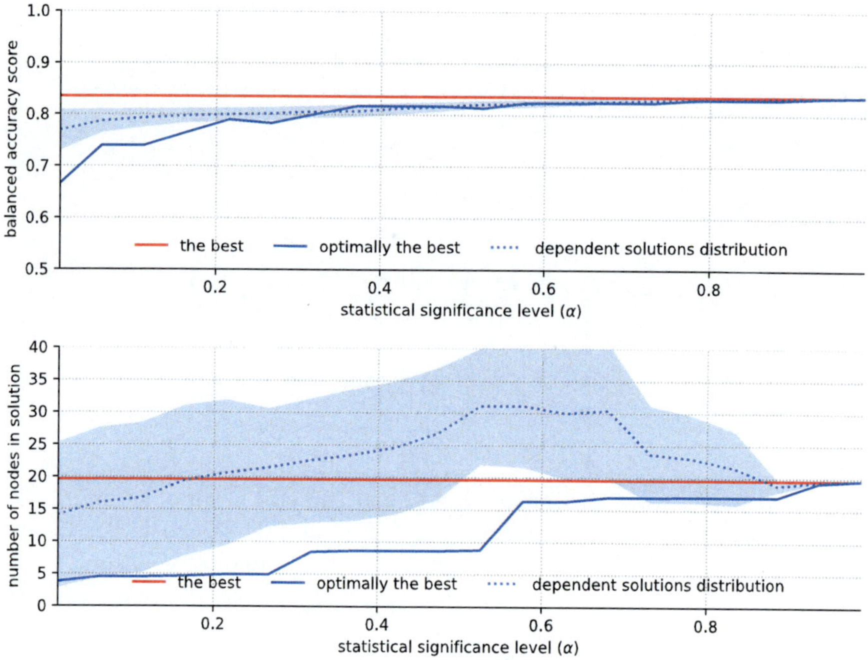

Fig. 2. Top – the relationship between the balanced accuracy of the model selected on the basis of the proposed method and α value in comparison to the best model in the hyperparameter review. Bottom – the relationship between the number of nodes in the selected models and α value. The results presented are the average of all folds. *The best* is the model with the highest *balanced accuracy* and *optimally the best* is the model selected based on the proposed method.

The results show that with the increase of α value, the average balanced accuracy of the models is getting closer and closer to the best model, although even with the small alpha there are no statistical differences between them, and at the same time the size of the tree, which is shown by the number of nodes, also increases. The choice of the optimal tree was based on selecting such a small value of alpha so that the size of the tree was as small as possible, but at the same time that this model would not deviate from the distribution of dependent solutions, i.e., that it would not be an outlier. Finally, it was decided to choose the value of alpha equal to 0.2, at which the tree size is reduced from 19.56 to 4.84 and the results are in the dependent solution deviation (balanced accuracy).

For models annotated as *the best* and *optimally the best* the confusion matrix was calculated and averaged across the fold (Fig. 3). The results show that despite minor differences, the group of suspects fares the worst. This is expected due to the complexity of this group, which, despite the presence of a glaucomatous optic disc, is not yet a glaucoma group.

Actual \ Predicted	C	G	S
C	11.68	0.12	2.00
G	0.20	12.44	1.36
S	1.88	1.48	11.04

Actual \ Predicted	C	G	S
C	11.92	0.24	1.64
G	0.76	10.84	2.40
S	3.96	1.04	9.40

Fig. 3. Confusion matrix for the best model in the full review (left) and optimally the best model selected on the basis of the proposed method with $\alpha = 0.2$ (right). *C – healthly controls, G – glaucoma patients, S – glaucoma suspects.*

5 Conclusions

This paper presents a method for selecting an interpretable model of decision trees for the classification of glaucoma, both developed as well as a group called glaucoma suspects. The models were trained on a set of data acquired from 211 patients and classified into glaucoma progression groups by an experienced ophthalmologist. The proposed method, by reviewing tree parameters and relying on statistical tests, obtained a balanced accuracy score of about 80% in the 3–class classification problem, which proves that in a fairly simple way this approach could preserve a high score *balanced accuracy* metric and simultaneously increase its interpretability of the model by reducing its size. Finally, the statistical significance level 0.2 was chosen, for which the dependent models were considered from the best based on the accuracy metric, and this allowed to reduce the size of the CART from average 19.56 to 4.84 nodes.

Acknowledgements. Special thanks to Paweł Ksieniewicz, from Wroclaw University of Science and Technology (WUST), for help in the described research and to D. Robert Iskander, also from WUST, for the guidance over the prepared manuscript.

Project supported by *InterDok – Interdisciplinary Doctoral Studies Projects* at Wroclaw University of Science and Technology, a project co-financed by the European Union under the European Social Fund, and by the Polish National Agency for Academic Exchange (NAWA, PPI/APM/2019/1/00085/DEC/1).

References

1. Quigley, H.A., Broman, A.T.: The number of people with glaucoma worldwide in 2010 and 2020. Br. J. Ophthalmol. **90**(3), 262–267 (2006)
2. Tatham, A.J., Medeiros, F.A., Zangwill, L.M., Weinreb, R.N.: Strategies to improve early diagnosis in glaucoma. In: Progress in Brain Research, vol. 221, pp. 103–133. Elsevier (2015)
3. Kim, J.-A., Kim, T.-W., Weinreb, R.N., Lee, E.J., Girard, M.J.A., Mari, J.M.: Lamina cribrosa morphology predicts progressive retinal nerve fiber layer loss in eyes with suspected glaucoma. Sci. Rep. **8**(1), 1–10 (2018)
4. Kurmann, T., et al.: Expert level automated biomarker identification in optical coherence tomography scans. Sci. Rep. **9**(1), 1–9 (2019)
5. Yow, A.P., et al.: Automated circumpapillary retinal nerve fiber layer segmentation in high-resolution swept-source oct. In: 2020 42nd Annual International Conference of the IEEE Engineering in Medicine Biology Society (EMBC), pp. 1832–1835 (2020)
6. Sułot, D., Alonso-Caneiro, D., Iskander, D.R., Collins, M.J.: Deep learning approaches for segmenting Bruch's membrane opening from OCT volumes. OSA Continuum **3**(12), 3351–3364 (2020)
7. Maetschke, S., Antony, B., Ishikawa, H., Wollstein, G., Schuman, J., Garnavi, R.: A feature agnostic approach for glaucoma detection in OCT volumes. PLoS One **14**(7), e0219126 (2019)
8. Ran, A.R., et al.: Deep learning in glaucoma with optical coherence tomography: a review. Eye **35**(1), 1–14 (2020)
9. Murtagh, P., Greene, G., O'Brien, C.: Current applications of machine learning in the screening and diagnosis of glaucoma: a systematic review and meta-analysis. Int. J. Ophthalmol. **13**(1), 149 (2020)
10. Weinreb, R.N., Khaw, P.T.: Primary open-angle glaucoma. The Lancet **363**(9422), 1711–1720 (2004)
11. Vellido, A.: The importance of interpretability and visualization in machine learning for applications in medicine and health care. Neural Comput. Appl. **32**(24), 18069–18083 (2019). https://doi.org/10.1007/s00521-019-04051-w
12. Kulikowski, C.A.: Pattern recognition approach to medical diagnosis. IEEE Trans. Syst. Sci. Cybern. **6**(3), 173–178 (1970)
13. Krzyżanowska-Berkowska, P., Czajor, K., Iskander, D.R.: Associating the biomarkers of ocular blood OW with lamina cribrosa parameters in normotensive glaucoma suspects. Comparison to glaucoma patients and healthy controls. PLoS One **16**(3), e0248851 (2021) (in review)
14. Loh, W.-Y.: Classification and regression trees. Wiley Interdisciplinary Rev. Data Min. Knowl. Disc. **1**(1), 14–23 (2011)
15. Pedregosa, F., et al.: Scikit-learn: machine learning in Python. J. Mach. Learn. Res. **12**, 2825–2830 (2011)
16. Tabachnick, B.G., Fidell, L.S.: Experimental designs using ANOVA. Thomson/Brooks/Cole Belmont, CA (2007)
17. Bergstra, J.S., Bardenet, R., Bengio, Y., Kegl, B.: Algorithms for hyper-parameter optimization. In: Advances in Neural Information Processing Systems, pp. 2546–2554 (2011)
18. Alpaydin, E.: Introduction to Machine Learning. MIT Press, Cambridge (2020)
19. Santafe, G., Inza, I., Lozano, J.A.: Dealing with the evaluation of supervised classification algorithms. Artif. Intell. Rev. **44**(4), 467–508 (2015). https://doi.org/10.1007/s10462-015-9433-y

Initial Results of Lower Limb Exoskeleton Therapy with Human Gait Analysis for a Paraplegic Patient

Luca Toth[1,2,3](✉), Adam Schiffer[3,4], Veronika Pinczker[1], Peter Muller[4], Andras Buki[1], and Peter Maroti[3]

[1] Neurosurgery Clinic, University of Pecs, Pecs, Hungary
[2] Medical School, Institute for Translational Medicine, University of Pecs, Pecs, Hungary
[3] 3D Printing Centre, University of Pecs, Pecs, Hungary
[4] Faculty of Engineering and Information Technology, University of Pecs, Pecs, Hungary

Abstract. Traumatic spinal cord injury (SCI) is a devastating condition affecting the young adult population. Complete SCI results in paraplegia, therefore, the patient is forced to use a wheelchair, withal mobility and activity of daily living is severely decreased. Recently, robotic lower limb exoskeletons have been utilized as a rehabilitation tool for SCI patients to improve the efficiency of the therapy, replace wheelchairs, and intended to reduce complications due to immobile lifestyle. According to our knowledge, there is no standardized protocol for exoskeleton therapy, furthermore, there is a need for objective evaluation of the efficiency of the therapy. In this work, our aim is to objectively evaluate the long-term impact of exoskeleton therapy on general health and rehabilitation therapy in a single case trial. The goal is to assess treatment accuracy by evaluating gait and stability parameters with our non-invasive movement analysis system along with general rehabilitation functional tests. Functional tests showed significant improvement after exoskeleton therapy. According to our results, there is a significant improvement in gait parameters, such as velocity and cadence, and a decrease in swing time following the rehabilitation program. The oscillation for stability analysis were decreased significantly in all planes and resulted in reduced wrist joint movement, justifying the stable hand use and improved balance. The markerless gait and stability analysis proves the importance of exoskeleton training in active rehabilitation therapy that resulted in significant improvement in balance and oscillation during the rehabilitation process. Although, the exact training protocol needs further investigation.

Keywords: Exoskeleton · Gait · Analysis · Functional test · SCI · Neurorehabilitation

N. Piaseczna et al. (Eds.): EMBS ICS 2020, AISC 1360, pp. 151–157, 2022.
https://doi.org/10.1007/978-3-030-88976-0_20

1 Introduction

Following a complete SCI lesion, the patients are forced to use wheelchairs, therefore, the activity of daily living as well as the quality of life is severely affected [1]. The prevalence of SCI is around 200.000 in the US, the incidence globally is almost 200.000/year, mainly affecting the young adult population, therefore rehabilitation therapy is essential [1–3]. In case of a complete lesion, robotic lower limb exoskeleton therapy aims to provide assistance for paralyzed patients, promotes the effect of therapy, and reduces the long-term complications related to immobilisation due to wheelchair use, such as osteoporosis, joint contractures, pressure sores or depression [1–3]. The effect of therapy is most frequently evaluated by observation of basic movement patterns visually by experts or physiotherapists, but the values are still subjective [4]. To materialize the rehabilitation results, gait analysis could be a viable tool however, the complex technical instrument impedes the objective data collection. Furthermore, the exoskeleton equipment hampers the precise analysis due to extensions such as crutches, robotic parts, etc. [2–4]. Accordingly, our aim was to objectively evaluate the rehabilitation outcomes in a single case trial according to functional rehabilitation measures, along with bone density as well as applying a self-developed complex non-marker gait analysis system, including spatiotemporal characterization of the oscillations of the spine base and limbs in the sagittal and coronal planes, along with wrist quiver analysis, due to the obligatory use of the crutches [6].

2 Materials and Methods

2.1 Patient Description, Training Protocol, and System Set Up

This study was approved by the Hungarian Medical Research Council (OGYÉI/48735/2017). Our 31-year-old patient suffered complete SCI injury on Th11 level, 2 years ago. According to the training protocol, before the robotic training, the team performed preparative physiotherapy to improve the trunk balance [1]. Afterwards, exoskeleton training was performed five days a week for six months by using a ReWalk P6.0 (ReWalk RoboticsTM Personal 6.0) robotic lower limb exoskeleton. The exoskeleton provides powered hip and knee motion to enable wheelchair-bound individuals to stand and walk again. The predefined settings provide the maximum amount of motor assistance to move the legs consistently through a predefined gait pattern. The patient controls the movement using subtle changes in the center of gravity. During therapy, the main functional turning points were indicated as milestones. General rehabilitation outcomes and movement analysis were performed in every milestone [1]. To evaluate posture changes, stability and to perform gait cycle analysis, a markerless measurement system was utilized, which consist of Kinect ONE sensor that is capable to transmit up to 11 data streams in real-time. The sensor is able to identify up to 6 persons with the skeleton model containing 25 connection joints for each body in the three-dimensional space. The developed MATLAB environment provides 25–30 frames per second (fps) recording speed. The operating range for the sensor measurements is between 0.4–4 m. Our software model encompasses high-speed recording, denoising, and signal processing that provides the stability parameters and gait cycle values. For the movement analysis, gait cycle test and stabilization analysis were performed at the milestones and the mean values of five different measurements are presented by wearing the exoskeleton device and using crutches, thus signal processing and prediction were exceptionally important to eliminate the harassing artefacts. Figure 1 shows the measurement setup with the 3D sensor that measures in the sagittal (S), coronal (C), and transverse (T) planes. The interface helps control the 3D sensor and the measurement, the PC is for real-time data recording and for post-processing.

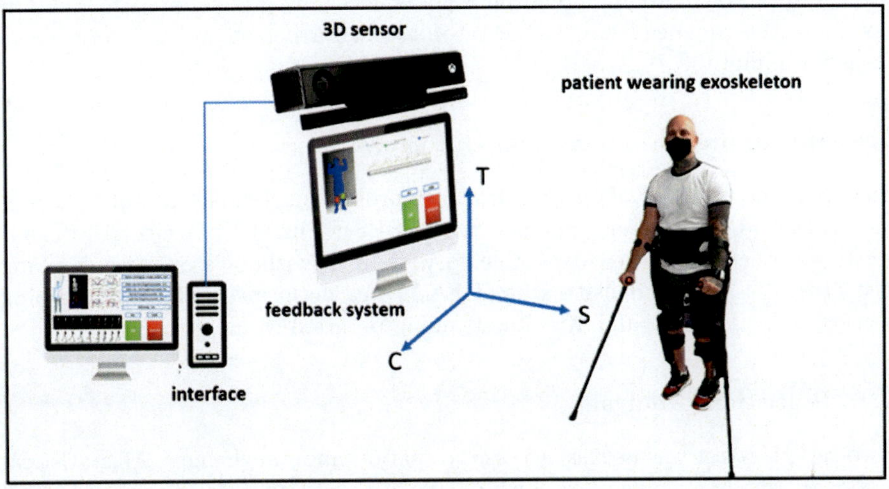

Fig. 1. The measurement setup with the 3D sensor measuring in the sagittal (S) coronal (C) and transverse (T) planes with our volunteer.

2.2 Gait and Stability Measurements

Spatial, angular, and temporal characteristics of gait and stability were measured at given milestones. As a first measurement, standing up on the device was analyzed. The damping of the oscillation of the spine base and wrists were measured and analyzed in the sagittal (S) and coronal (C) planes. The transverse plane (T) supports the calculation of the first time point after standing up. The excursion is calculated from the standard deviation in cm of the joint. For the stability analysis, the subject was asked to stand up and remain standing for 10 s until the balance equilibrium was reached. For the gait analysis, the patient was asked to walk in a pathway 7 m long wearing the exoskeleton. Transient movements occurred at the first 3 m therefore, the analyzed data refers to the steady state phase thereafter.

As the joint trajectories were sampled 30 Hz, the stability and gait cycle analysis were maintainable with sufficient accuracy. The coordinates in all planes of the measured joints were low-pass filtered with a fourth-order Butterworth filter. The dropped or covered joints during the measurement were predicted by Kalman filter. The gait cycle events, i.e., heel strike (HS), toe-off (TO), and middle swing (MS), are calculated from the spatial and angular joint data curves. For the exoskeleton-assisted gait analysis, we validated our algorithm by comparing it with the timing of the same gait events during the gait cycle. By detecting the gait phases (stride and stance), the stride interval and stride length could be calculated for the complete gait cycle. As the step length indicates the distance from a specific stance-phase event of one foot to the same event of the other foot, stride length is the distance from the initial contact of one foot to the following initial contact of the same foot. The calculated velocity refers to the average speed of the body along the S plane in meters per second. The analysis results in the cadence, that is, the rate at which a person walks, expressed in steps per minute [6,7].

2.3 Rehabilitation Functional Outcomes

To access the progress of the functional improvement Trunk Control Measurement Scale (TCMS), Berg Balance Scale (BBS), Timed Up'n Go test (TUG) was used, once the patient was able to walk 10 m without stop, 10 m walking test (10 mWT). Bone density scan (DEXA) was performed before the walking section of the training and after the training program (6 months).

2.4 Statistical Analysis

Two-sample t-test was used to access the spatio-temporal changes. All statistical tests had the significance level of $p < 0.05$. All statistics were performed using Origin Pro 2018 software.

3 Results

3.1 Spatiotemporal Characteristics

Before and after the rehabilitation process, a significant improvement of gait parameters were observed, including velocity and cadence, and a decrease in swing time. The step length cannot be improved because it is determined by the exoskeleton settings. The oscillation for stability analysis is measured by the spine base joint deviation in the steady state in S and C planes. Table 1 shows the results of the spine base (SB) and the left wrist (LW) oscillation as its standard deviation in two planes at the beginning and the end of the rehabilitation process. According to the results, the oscillation significantly decreased in the sagittal and coronal planes as well, resulting in reduced wrist joint movement, justifying the stable hand use and improved balance.

Table 1. Oscillation standard (std) deviation results of standing up measured in coronal and sagittal planes. Significant values are marked bold ($p < 0.05$). 3 measurements (3/1,3/2,3/3) were performed at the beginning and at the end of the therapy as well.

Joint	Beginning (std. deviation)			End (std. deviation)			t-test value
	Meas. 3/1	Meas. 3/2	Meas. 3/3	Meas. 3/1	Meas. 3/2	Meas. 3/3	
SB_C	4.68	1.45	4.17	0.41	0.18	0.42	**0.037**
SB_S	2.50	1.29	3.25	0.31	0.64	0.14	**0.028**
LW_C	7.94	7.37	7.38	2.87	0.42	0.60	**0.017**
LW_S	3.36	5.39	3.33	1.98	1.15	0.99	**0.024**

Figure 2(a) presents the steady state spine base oscillation in the sagittal and coronal planes at the beginning (blue) and end (red) of the rehabilitation. Figure 2(b) shows how the wrist oscillation changes at the beginning (blue) and end (red) of the rehabilitation process. During gait analysis, the cadence significantly increased from 45.5/min to 60.2/min over the rehabilitation period.

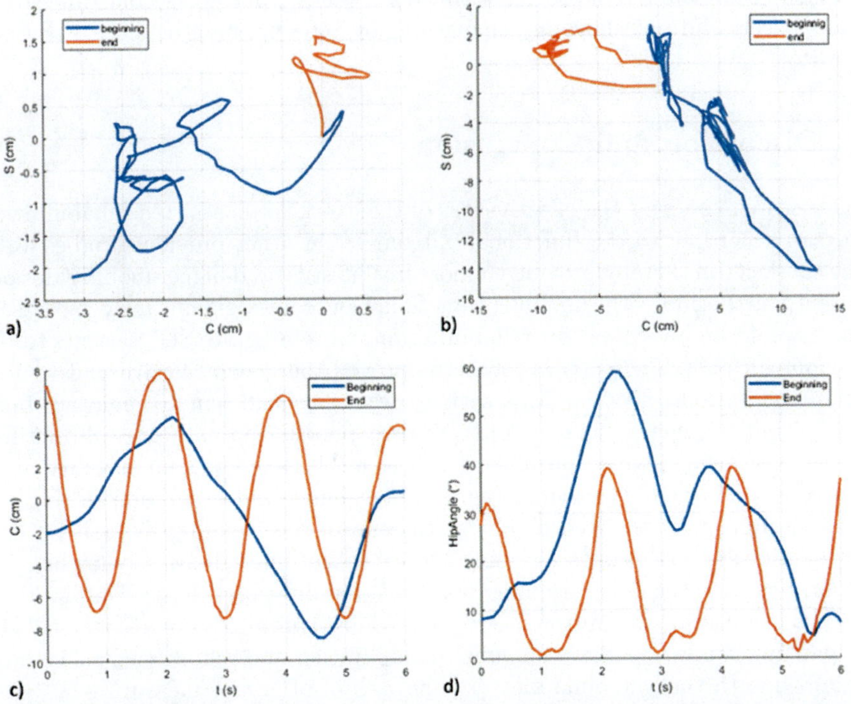

Fig. 2. Steady state oscillation in sagittal (S) and coronal (C) planes at the beginning and end of the rehabilitation process of (a) spine base (b) right wrist; (c) Periodical spine base oscillation during the walking test in coronal plane; (d) The angle of the hip during the walking test.

There was no significant increase in the step length (from 1.00 m to 1.06 m). The gait speed is changed from 0.38 m/s to 0.53 m/s throughout the training. The swinging phases of the gait cycle were decreased from 41% to 37% and the stance phase increased from 59% to 63% during therapy. Figure 2(c) illustrates the spine base oscillation in the coronal plane before and after the rehabilitation. The oscillation of the spine base significantly decreased from 5.3 sec to 2.1 sec. The main difference with the increase in frequency was that the oscillations along the coronal plane became much more uniform by the end of rehabilitation. The spine base showed a sinusoidal and rhythmic wave in a range about 10–15 cm in walking. Figure 2(d) shows the hip angle periodic oscillation during walking. The amplitude of the hip angle is significantly lower at the end of the training protocol, and the curve is reasonably homogenous.

3.2 Rehabilitation Functional Outcomes

According to the functional rehabilitation outcomes, Trunk Control Measurement Scale, Berg Balance scale outcome considerably improved according to the baseline and to milestone measurement as well. The 10 m walking test performance significantly improved within two weeks from the second milestone. Bone density did not show any changes following a six months' active training protocol.

4 Discussion and Conclusion

Our research confirms the effectiveness of the exoskeleton assisted rehabilitation process, according to the functional outcomes and other previous studies [2,3]. The exoskeleton therapy provided a more free lifestyle and bigger mobility for our patient, furthermore the mobility functional outcomes significantly increased, which would be important for rehabilitation and reintegrate SCI patients to the previous lifestyle. The active protocol improved the general health and wellbeing of the patient, however, this activity was only sufficient to maintain bone density, but not increasing consequently, osteoporosis and pathological fractures as the main concerns remain unsolved. The markerless gait and stability analysis resulted in significant improvement in balance and oscillation during the rehabilitation process. Accordingly, at the end of the training, the gait pattern and spatio-temporal values resembled to a healthy individuals', confirming the importance of exoskeleton training in active rehabilitation therapy. Despite that, the main limitation is still the lack of a universal training protocol personalized for patient groups to achieve maximal rehabilitation and reduce medical complications due to the immobile lifestyle, the lack of objective measuring systems, and the price of novel exoskeleton devices. Our research presents initial data which could be a source for developing further training protocols and spatiotemporal analysis.

Acknowledgements. This work was supported by the Thematic Excellence Program 2020 – National Excellence Sub-program; Biomedical Engineering Project ("2020-4.1.1-TKP2020") of the University of Pecs, and National Economic Development and Innovation Program for Neurorehabilitation and Human-Machine Interface Developments [grant number GINOP-2.3.3-15-2016-00032].

References

1. Tóth, L., et al.: Rehabilitation of traumatic spinal cord injury with lower limb exoskeleton. Orvosi. Hetilap. **161**(29), 1200–1207 (2020)
2. Talaty, M., Esquenazi, A., Briceño, J.E.: Differentiating ability in users of the ReWalkTM powered exoskeleton. In: 2013 IEEE International Conference on Rehabilitation Robotics (2013)
3. Khan, A.S., et al.: Retraining walking over ground in a powered exoskeleton after spinal cord injury: a prospective cohort study to examine functional gains and neuroplasticity. J. NeuroEng. Rehabil. **16**, 145 (2019)
4. Muller, P., Schiffer, A.: Human gait cycle analysis using Kinect V2 sensor. Pollack Periodica **15**(3), 3–14 (2020)
5. Coutts, F.: Gait analysis in the therapeutic environment. Manual Therapy **4**(1), 2–10 (1999)
6. Ramanujam, A., et al.: Neuromechanical adaptations during a robotic powered exoskeleton assisted walking session. J. Spinal Cord Med. **45**(5), 518–528 (2017)
7. Buesing, C., et al.: Effects of a wearable exoskeleton stride management assist system (SMA®) on spatiotemporal gait characteristics in individuals after stroke: a randomized controlled trial. J. NeuroEng. Rehabil. **12**(69), 1–14 (2015)

Author Index

N. Piaseczna et al. (Eds.): EMBS ICS 2020, AISC 1360, pp. 159–160, 2022.
https://doi.org/10.1007/978-3-030-88976-0